KU-300-651

WITHDRAWN
HEALTH LIBRARY AT COUNTY

CLINICAL TRIALS

Edited by

Lelia Duley and Barbara Farrell

POSTGRADUATE MEDICAL CENTRE

PGMC LIBRARY
STAFFORD DGH
WESTON ROAD
STAFFORD ST16 3S∕

POSTGRADUATE MEDICAL LIBRARY
Cannock Community Hospital
Brunswick Road
CANNOCK   WS11 2XY
Tel (0785) 57731 Ext 4633

BMJ
Books

15·95

© BMJ Books 2002
BMJ Books is an imprint of the BMJ Publishing Group

All rights reserved. No part of this publication may be
reproduced, stored in a retrieval system, or transmitted, in any
form or by any means, electronic, mechanical, photocopying,
recording and/or otherwise, without the prior written
permission of the publishers.

First published in 2002
by BMJ Books, BMA House, Tavistock Square,
London WC1H 9JR

www.bmjbooks.com

British Library Cataloguing in Publication Data

A catalogue record for this book is available from the British Library

ISBN 0 7279 1599 1

Typeset by SIVA Math Setters, Chennai, India
Printed and bound in Spain by GraphyCems, Navarra

Contents

Contributors

Clive Adams
Academic Unit of Psychiatry
and Behavioural Sciences
University of Leeds

John Bell
Nuffield Department of Medicine
John Radcliffe Hospital
Oxford

Eivind Berge
Department of Clinical Neurosciences
Western General Hospital
Edinburgh

David A Braunholtz
Department of Public Health and Epidemiology
University of Birmingham

Mike Clarke
UK Cochrane Centre
NHS R&D Programme
Oxford

Carl E Counsell
Department of Clinical Neurosciences
University of Edinburgh

Richard Doll
ICRF/MRC/BHF Clinical Trial Service Unit and
Epidemiological Studies Unit
Radcliffe Infirmary
Oxford

Lelia Duley
Resource Centre for Randomised Trials
Institute of Health Sciences
Oxford

Barbara Farrell
Resource Centre for Randomised Trials
Institute of Health Sciences
Oxford

William J Gillespie
Dunedin School of Medicine
University of Otago
New Zealand

Adrian M Grant
Health Services Research Unit
University of Aberdeen

Richard J Lilford
Department of Public Health and Epidemiology
University of Birmingham

Ann Oakley
Social Science Research Unit
University of London
Institute of Education
London

Robin J Prescott
Medical Statistics Unit
University of Edinburgh

Susan Ross
Mount Sinai Hospital
Samuel Lunenfeld Research Institute and
Department of Health Administration
Toronto
Canada

Ian T Russell
Department of Health Sciences
University of York

Peter Sandercock
Department of Clinical Neurosciences
Western General Hospital
Edinburgh

Trevor Sheldon
Department of Health Sciences
University of York

Patsy Spark
Resource Centre for Randomised Trials
Institute of Health Sciences
Oxford

Hazel Thornton
Honorary Visiting Fellow
Department of Epidemiology and Public Health
University of Leicester

José Villar
World Health Organisation
Americas Region Special Programme
Programme of Research Development and Research
Training in Human Reproduction
Geneva

Charles Warlow
Department of Clinical Neurosciences
Western General Hospital
University of Edinburgh

Foreword

The systematic evaluation of clinical interventions using clinical trials has provided the foundation for rationally applied health care in the modern era. The methodology that underlies this activity has evolved dramatically over the past thirty years to provide an increasingly robust system for establishing, with statistical support, the role of specific therapeutic interventions. In this age of evidence-based medicine and meta-analysis, it is important to remember that all these novel approaches rely on a foundation of clinical trials.

This book provides an important framework for those applying and developing clinical trial methodology. It provides reviews on current trial methodology, focusing on specific issues that challenge trialists and those attempting to implement the results of trials. In particular, it raises important issues for trialists going forward. Specifically, several challenges remain unresolved and present significant tests for trialists; the application of this methodology to chronic, non-fatal diseases has not been uniformly successful. Similarly, the availability of large sets of agents for individual diseases, such as multiple new therapies for HIV and transplantation, presents a challenge to classical clinical trial design. The recognition that patients differ individually in their response to therapy based on genetic variation (pharmacogenetics), will provide additional challenges to existing methodologies and opportunities to make trials even more powerful in less heterogeneous patient subsets.

This book sets the stage for what remains a remarkably exciting and dynamic field. Our ability to evaluate rigorously what we do clinically remains the essence of modern biomedicine.

John Bell

Preface

Randomised trials are well established as providing the most reliable evidence to guide clinical decision making. As the demand for reliable evidence grows, more and more people are getting involved in doing trials. Many others are wondering how to get started. In September 2000 the Resource Centre for Randomised Trials organised a one-day meeting which aimed to share ideas, experiences and visions for the future of clinical trials. The chapters in this book are based on presentations at that meeting.

We hope the book will be of interest to anyone involved in trials. The chapters cover a range of topics, but the main theme of the book is promoting understanding and sharing of expertise in the conduct and management of high quality trials.

Lelia Duley and Barbara Farrell

Acknowledgements

We are grateful for the tremendous support we have received in the preparation of this book. Particular thanks to the chapter authors, for rapid delivery of their contributions, and to the participants at the meeting upon which the book is based. Thanks also to Nina Armstrong, Barbara Roberts, Mary Tivnan, and Liza Wang at the Resource Centre for Randomised Trials.

Chief thanks for *The Cochrane Controlled Trials Register* go to all those members of the Cochrane Collaboration who have played a role in its development and maintenance.

The review on which much of Chapter 6 was based was funded by a grant from the United Kingdom Research and Development, Health Technology Assessment Programme. The chapter authors are grateful to the study's research associates, Sandra Kiauka and Iain Colthart without whom the review could not have been undertaken, and to Daphne Russell and Sue Shepherd who contributed to the original report.

1 Comparing like with like and the development of randomisation–goodbye anecdotes

CHARLES WARLOW

"During the last five and twenty years I have never failed to treat successfully the most inveterate and severe cases of migraine by the introduction of an ordinary tape seton through the skin at the back of the neck". So wrote Walter Whitehead, a Manchester surgeon, in the *British Medical Journal* a century ago.[1] Needless to say tape setons do not get a mention in *The Cochrane Library*![2] Indeed, even the most elderly clinician would probably not know that this involves passing a piece of ordinary household tape through a fold of skin at the back of the neck, and then inviting the patient to slide it from side to side, every day for three months. The treatment has vanished, not because it was properly evaluated and found to be useless, but because fashions changed.

Treatments based on theory and anecdote without being properly tested inevitably give way to the next fashionable theory, and more anecdotes. A hundred years ago, there was no medical culture of comparing the results of one treatment with another, or with no treatment, in an organised way. Hardly anyone thought it necessary to form two comparable groups of patients; with one group being given one treatment and the other group the other, or no treatment, to "control" for biases. The biases that arise from making inferences based on the outcomes of single, several or even hundreds of patients treated with something that was supposed to work. The plural of anecdote clearly is not data. And certainly no one at the time was advocating randomising patients so that reliably comparable groups could be formed which would be so similar in all known, and unknown ways, that any definite difference in their outcomes could be assumed to be due to the difference in their treatment.

1

The first randomised controlled trial was published little more than 50 years ago.[3] In this trial, the statistician Austin Bradford Hill persuaded the doctors to randomly allocate patients with pulmonary tuberculosis to either streptomycin or no treatment, partly as a way of distributing fairly the small supply of streptomycin then available, as well as finding out if it worked. Probably no one would now be able to ration treatment in this rather sensible way, although it has been suggested when a licensed treatment is expensive and uncertain in its effect and where some patients receive it and others don't in the uncontrolled muddle of routine clinical practice. So called postcode prescribing. Paradoxically, many opposed to postcode prescribing also, irrationally, support the notion of local autonomy rather than centralised decisions for the delivery of health care

It is now widely accepted that the most efficient method to evaluate a therapeutic intervention, whether old and never tested or new and untested, is by comparing two groups of patients who are so similar at baseline that their outcomes only differ by chance, or because one group received an effective or harmful therapeutic intervention. And that the best way to construct such groups is by random allocation, without the treating clinician being able to predict which group a patient is going to be in.[4] The scientific, and so clinical advantages, of randomisation have taken a secure hold on medical thinking and, as discussed in the next chapter, there are presently about one third of a million reports of randomised or possibly randomised trials in *The Cochrane Library*.[2]

Bigger is usually better

In the early days of clinical trials, randomisation to control for the biases in evaluating treatments that can arise when patients receive one treatment or another on the whim of the treating clinician was too often regarded as enough. Frequently no consideration was given to the *precision* of the estimate of the treatment effect size, which depends on the number of patients with an outcome event and so on the number of randomised patients, and on the size of the treatment effect itself. Reliably finding modest treatment effects requires a surprising number of patients, particularly if the outcome to be avoided is not very common.[4] In small trials where there was "no statistically significant treatment effect" the conclusion was often drawn that there really was no treatment effect at all. Of course, such a "negative" result may just be due to bad luck and too much emphasis on a P value of more than 0.05, rather than to any real lack of treatment effect. The widespread use of confidence intervals to demonstrate the range of where the true treatment effect might lie is a relatively recent development.[5] There was, and sometimes still is, confusion between "no evidence of benefit" (where there may actually be a benefit but the trial is too small or badly designed to show it) and "evidence of no benefit" (where the trial is large enough and well designed enough to reasonably exclude a treatment effect size of clinical importance).

The development of meta-analysis in the 1970s by Tom Chalmers, Richard Peto, Iain Chalmers and others provided a method, but not a complete alternative, to effectively increase the overall sample size. Meta-analysis combines the results of several trials of the same intervention, provided the outcomes are similar enough across the trials and all or at least most of the trials can be found.[6,7] This literally "saved" the premature rejection of thrombolysis for acute myocardial infarction. From the late 1950s there had been a series of small and mostly "negative" randomised trials and the treatment was generally thought not to work. But, in the early 1980s, meta-analysis showed that there probably was a reduction in case fatality.[8,9] At the time meta-analysis was new and mistrusted more than it is now and so, although the clinical community was not convinced enough to change their clinical practice, they were prepared to randomise thousands of patients in what were the first "mega-trials" involving thousands rather than hundreds of patients, GISSI 1 and ISIS 2.[10,11] These trials were large enough to confirm the results of the meta-analysis, and thrombolysis is now standard treatment for acute myocardial infarction. The ethical dilemmas this presented to members of the data monitoring committee are discussed by Richard Doll (Chapter 8).

Almost the same story can be told for stroke units versus care within standard general medical wards. Before Peter Langhorne published his first meta-analysis of the small and mostly "negative" trials in 1993[12] hardly anyone believed that stroke units improved outcome after acute stroke. In this case the meta-analysis was convincing enough by itself to change clinical practice, no really large trials have ever been done, and stroke units are now regarded as an essential part of high quality care. Indeed, the National Service Framework for Older People in England and Wales mandates that by 2002 "Every general hospital that cares for people with stroke will have plans to introduce a specialised stroke service ..... from 2004".[13]

Miscellaneous problems and biases

But, even large randomised trials, and meta-analyses of similar trials, are not enough by themselves. There are important problems and biases to be considered.

Outcome selection and assessment

Outcomes must be selected carefully. For example, death alone is not adequate in trials of treatment for acute stroke, some measurement of disability and even quality of life in the many survivors is needed as well. Furthermore, treatment may have no effect on an outcome that is very obvious and easily measured by the trialists, but it may still be helpful in other ways. For example, a treatment may not prevent the spread of breast cancer but it might have a big effect on other outcomes more difficult to measure but of great concern to patients, such as pain.

It is best if people who are "blind" to the treatment allocation assess outcome, so they cannot be influenced by any conscious or unconscious bias in favour of or against the treatment being assessed. This applies particularly to "softer" outcomes like pain or fatigue, rather than "harder" outcomes such as death. But, even though the fact of death cannot be disputed, the cause of death can be incorrect if there is observer bias in the categorisation process. This is why trials often have a separate committee, blinded if possible to treatment allocation, to evaluate important outcomes in individual patients.

Blinding patients

The importance of "blinding" the patients to which treatment they are taking, and so avoiding the effect on outcome of patient expectations, has been recognised for years. When the treatments are drugs this is easy, if expensive, to achieve with the use of placebos. It is not so easy when the trial is of surgery versus no surgery, although it is still possible and ideally even necessary. For example, it can be done, by anaesthesia and a skin incision and then the surgical procedure, or not, without the patient being aware of the choice. This was done in the trial which showed that internal mammary artery ligation did not improve angina.[14]

For evaluation of acupuncture it is possible to have a sham treatment by using the needles in the wrong place and in the wrong way, and for psychotherapy it is perhaps possible to "blind" the patient by having a comparison group of just non-specific counselling. But, often one has to accept that the patient will know the treatment and allowance is then made in the choice and assessment of outcomes.

Publication and lag time bias

It is no good doing trials and meta-analyses, and then not disseminating the results quickly. It is surely unethical to invite the collaboration of patients in clinical trials and then to not use the information gained for the public good. Moreover, trials with "positive" results tend to see the light of day rather quicker than those with "negative" results. Negative trials may never be published at all, so biasing the literature. Clinical behaviour is then not appropriate because relevant data have been suppressed.[15]

Subgroup analysis

Clinicians always want to know what to do with their individual patients; treat this one who will benefit, and not that one who will be harmed. However, statisticians argue that randomised trials generally provide an "on average" result so that if similar patients to the trial patients are treated with something proven in a positive trial there will be net benefit. Some patients may be harmed but more will benefit, the greatest good for the greatest number. Between these extremes lies the identification of a few particular types of patients, or subgroups, and the analysis of the treatment effect in them may be of interest, for example old versus young, severe versus mild disease. Such subgroup analyses are fraught with difficulty because treatment effects can easily emerge by chance in subgroups which are always, by definition, smaller than the entire trial.[16,17] The more subgroups there are, the bigger the problem. Being misled by chance findings in this way is particularly likely if the overall trial result is negative.

To get partially around this difficulty it is generally best for any subgroups of potential interest to be defined at the trial design stage. This is both so that they can be properly identified from the baseline data, and so that the trialist cannot be accused of data dredging after the overall trial result is known. Even better is to regard subgroup analysis as hypothesis generating, and then to confirm the results in an independent trial. This means that more than one trial of an intervention has to be done at about the same time, as was the case for example with carotid surgery[18,19] and acute ischaemic stroke.[20]

Generalisability

Many argue that the results of a randomised trial in a group of patients can only be applied to precisely the same sort of patients in future clinical practice. This requires the trial patients to be well described (for example by age, sex, and severity of illness), which is easy and reasonable. But, it does not require every single eligible patient to be randomised. Nor does it require any non-randomised but eligible patients to be described and followed up, which is hugely complicated and therefore expensive, and seldom complete. For future practice, the inference from a trial comes from the results in the randomised, not the non-randomised patients, and this is applied to *similar* patients in the future, not *all* patients, and never precisely the same sort of patients as were in the trial.

Generalising a trial result to patients in the future does require common sense in how far one goes. It is generally reasonable to apply the results to perhaps slightly older patients than went into the trial, provided there is unlikely to be a problem with adverse treatment effects in this age group, which should be reasonably easy to predict from observational studies. It might not be sensible, however, to give thrombolytic treatment to an acute ischaemic stroke patient too far beyond three hours from symptom onset (where the trials were generally negative) because it is conceivable that the risk of haemorrhagic transformation of a mature infarct then outweighs any benefit.[21] So in designing a randomised trial it is important to have fairly broad entry criteria to cover the range of patients likely to benefit, to describe quite carefully what the patients looked like at baseline, and to do a few a priori defined subgroup analyses with considerable caution.[4]

Obstacles to randomised trials

If one accepts that randomised trials really are presently the best way of evaluating therapeutic interventions, old untested ones as well as new, then various obstacles have to be overcome.

Ethical concerns

There is undoubtedly an ethical difficulty if randomised trials are regarded merely as experimentation on human beings, without gain and even with possible harm for the individuals concerned, notwithstanding their consent which may be more coerced than informed in some situations. Even if the greater good will be served by well conducted trials (in the sense of benefiting future patients), this is not necessarily good enough for an individual being asked to enter a trial. That person wants to know "What's in it for me?" and "What are the alternatives?"

At one level some regard the altruistic act of entering a trial as sufficient justification for a patient's participation, provided the individual concerned is fully aware of the choice he or she is making. But, in addition, entering a trial may well be a selfish act, because by so doing the patient will almost certainly get better care than in ordinary clinical practice.[22] For example, the trial treatments are carefully thought about by many experts, including grant-giving bodies, and an ethics committee. They are not given on the whim of an individual clinician. The patients in a trial are likely to be very carefully diagnosed, monitored efficiently, systematically treated along guidelines, and followed up rigorously. Attention will be paid to any other illnesses, or complications of the presenting illness, by collaborators who are likely to be well informed about that illness, and certainly in close contact with the trial organisers who will be particularly expert. And, of course, the results are likely to be kept under review by an independent data monitoring committee who will alert the trial organisers if definite harm or benefit is established. This is a far cry from the hurly burly of routine clinical practice. It is hardly surprising that patients in clinical trials, even those allocated the control treatment, tend to do better than expected.[22] Interestingly, even in the very first randomised trial, the control patients with pulmonary tuberculosis had the advantage of being given the highest priority for admission for the conventional treatment of the time.

The alternative to randomisation is for the patient to take one or other of the treatments being compared. But which one? If the clinician is genuinely uncertain which treatment to recommend then the best option for the patient must be to be randomised. This way, at the very least, half the patients will avoid some unexpected adverse effect of the new treatment, and often the old treatment has turned out to be the best option.[23] A recent example is the randomised trial of implantation of fetal cells into the brain of patients with Parkinson's disease. Although there may have been a small benefit after a year, some patients allocated this treatment developed a completely unforeseen and intractable movement disorder a few years later. Most unfortunately, some untreated control patients were *not* protected from this adverse effect, because they were offered the surgical implantation at the end of the first year.[24]

Of course individual clinician, and patient, uncertainty is a crucial prerequisite. If a clinician is certain, for whatever reason, that a treatment must be given to an individual patient then it is unethical to seek their consent to randomisation to the possibility of not getting that treatment. If the clinician is certain, for whatever reason, that the treatment should *not* be given, then it is unethical for the patient to be randomised to that treatment. But, if the clinician is genuinely uncertain and can share this uncertainty with the patient, then it becomes not just ethical to randomise but also in the patient's best interest because the trial will probably provide the best care.[22,25] It will also provide the best science because the clinician will have the treatment question answered for precisely the type of patients he or she is uncertain about. Naturally not all clinicians are uncertain about exactly the same patients but at least if their uncertainties overlap, a group of clinicians can randomise a wide range of patients and so explore a number of subgroups of interest and maximise generalisability of the trial results.

To facilitate randomised trials it is extremely important that patients, the public at large, and particularly ethics committees, understand these principles and what the alternatives are: unfettered, non-randomised experimentation on unsuspecting patients exposed to huge variations in clinical practice, crazed treatments based on unsubstantiated theory and the results of the last case, or maybe no treatment at all even though this might very well be appropriate.

Bureaucracy

Throughout modern society there is a most unfortunate tendency for a proliferation of red tape. Everything has to be monitored, often repeatedly, every back has to be guarded against all possible contingencies. This is not just a problem in medical research but also in routine medical practice, for teachers, the police, social workers, and many others. This red tape can very easily strangle research by making it just too exhausting to do. And so the young researcher gives up and retreats into private practice, and the old researcher takes early retirement or becomes an administrator. Society at large has got to reverse this trend. If not, the cost in terms of investigator time and reams of paper will soon exceed the cost of the occasional problem, if it hasn't already.

Practical concerns

There are clearly practical difficulties in running and contributing to randomised trials. Everyone is busy, more so than ever it seems.

Routine clinical practice consumes all the time there is, and the red tape consumes even more. So if trials are to be done in routine clinical practice, from where the therapeutic questions are derived and where the patients are for recruitment into trials, they must be part of the routine culture. The expectation should be that clinicians do trials as part of their job, and for that they must be properly funded. In the United Kingdom, the National Health Service must do research, not just care for patients and in the last few years a modest start has been made with the Health Technology Assessment Programme.

There must also be slick trial organisation that really works. Naturally trials would become more part of clinical practice if they were streamlined and straightforward to do, without pages and pages of forms to fill in and over intrusive external monitoring.

Lack of resources

Finally, trials cost money. They do not need to cost as much as many of the pharmaceutical industry trials, where an extraordinary amount of information and monitoring is demanded (often unnecessarily). Nevertheless, they can still be expensive. But, if they did become streamlined enough to be part of routine clinical practice, with minimal but sufficient data collection, they would be less expensive. In any event, the cost of *not* doing trials and allowing potentially toxic and expensive treatments into routine clinical practice is surely inappropriate. It is also inappropriate to devolve all trials to the pharmaceutical industry. Not only may there be conflict of interest and delayed or no publication of trials with negative results, but there will be no evaluation of interventions which are of no interest to the industry, such as surgical treatments, rehabilitation techniques, and non-patented drugs.

Conclusions

Until someone thinks of a better way, randomised controlled trials will remain the best and most efficient way of assessing most therapeutic interventions. Of course, there are some situations where trials are impractical and so less persuasive non-randomised comparisons have to do. For example, it would hardly be possible to randomly allocate individuals to a public health campaign to improve their diet without that same campaign influencing the control individuals to change their diet too. Indeed, because of this problem of "contamination", it was impossible to conduct a convincing trial of anti-smoking advice, at least with a sufficient sample size to show any definite effect on the prevention of vascular events. Too many of those randomised to quitting advice did not quit, and too many of those randomised to no intervention decided to quit.[26]

Just because randomised trials are the best method does not mean they cannot be improved, for example by standardising their reporting.[27] We need to be constantly making trials better as various new problems and biases come to light, and we must constantly be making the statistical analyses more robust without being so complicated that clinicians and policy makers cannot understand them. Simple is usually best, particularly if any complicated alternative analysis leads to precisely the same conclusion. But to do trials at all does require the right milieu. Clinicians, health managers, and politicians have to be convinced of their utility and that there is no sensible alternative. The general public have to realise this too. We have to educate people so they understand the purpose of randomisation and why sample sizes need to be so large. We must educate clinicians that inappropriate subgroup analyses can lead to hopelessly flawed conclusions and damaging changes in clinical practice. We must persuade the public that randomised trials are not making guinea pigs out of sick people but are the best way of helping sick people in general, now and in the future. And, at the end of the day, funders of health services have to realise that the cost of *not* doing trials will probably be higher than doing them. Introducing new, untested treatments into routine care is not only expensive if they don't work, but the adverse effects will damage patients, and sometimes even kill patients. Funders of services must therefore be prepared to fund research to improve those services. At the same time, those who do randomised trials have a responsibility to do them well, to get the right answer, and to widely disseminate the results as quickly as possible.

References

1 Whitehead W. The surgical treatment of migraine. *BMJ* 1901;i:335–6.
2 Cochrane Collaboration. *Cochrane Library*. Issue 2. Oxford: Update Software, 2001.
3 Medical Research Council. Streptomycin in Tuberculous Trials Committee. Streptomycin treatment of pulmonary tuberculous. *BMJ* 1948;ii:769–82.

4 Collins R, MacMahon S. Reliable assessment of the effects of treatment on mortality and major morbidity. 1: clinical trials. *Lancet* 2001;**357**:373–80.

5 Shakespeare TP, Gebski VJ, Veness MJ, Simes J. Improving interpretation of clinical studies by use of confidence levels, clinical significance curves, and risk-benefit contours. *Lancet* 2001;**357**:1349–53.

6 Pogue J, Yusuf S. Overcoming the limitations of current meta-analysis of randomised controlled trials. *Lancet* 1998;**351**:47–52.

7 Lau J, Ioannidis JPA, Schmid CH. Summing up evidence: one answer is not always enough. *Lancet* 1998;**351**:123–7.

8 Stampfer MJ, Goldhaber SZ, Yusuf S, Peto R, Hennekens CH. Effect of intravenous streptokinase on acute myocardial infarction. *N Engl J Med* 1982;**307**:1180–2.

9 Yusuf S, Collins R, Peto R, *et al.* Intravenous and intracoronary fibrinolytic therapy in acute myocardial infarction: overview of results on mortality, reinfarction and side-effects from 33 randomised controlled trials. *Eur Heart J* 1985;**6**:556–85.

10 Gruppo Italiano Per Lo Studio Della Streptochinasi Nell'infarto Miocardico (GISSI). Effectiveness of intravenous thrombolytic treatment in acute myocardial infarction. *Lancet* 1986;**i**:397–401.

11 ISIS-2 (Second International Study of Infarct Survival) Collaborative Group. Randomised trial of intravenous streptokinase, oral aspirin, both, or neither among 17,187 cases of suspected acute myocardial infarction: ISIS-2. *Lancet* 1988,**ii**:349–60.

12 Langhorne P, Williams BO, Gilchrist W, Howie K. Do stroke units save lives? *Lancet* 1993;**342**:395–8.

13 The National Service Framework for Older People. www.doh.gov.uk/nsf/olderpeople.htm (accessed 11 Jul 2001).

14 Cobb LA, Thomas GI, Dillard DH, Merendino KA, Bruce RA. An evaluation of internal-mammary-artery ligation by a double-blind technic. *N Engl J Med* 1959;**260**:1115–18.

15 Chalmers I. Underreporting research is scientific misconduct. *JAMA* 1990;**263**:1405–8.

16 Counsell CE, Clarke MJ, Slattery J, Sandercock PAG. The miracle of DICE therapy for acute stroke: fact or fictional product subgroup analysis. *BMJ* 1994;**309**:1677–81.

17 Assmann SF, Pocock SJ, Enos LE, Kasten LE. Subgroup analysis and other (mis)uses of baseline data in clinical trials. *Lancet* 2000;**355**:1064–9.

18 European Carotid Surgery Trialists' Collaborative Group. Randomised trial of endarterectomy for recently symptomatic carotid stenosis: final results of the MRC European Carotid Surgery Trial (ECST). *Lancet* 1998;**351**:1379–87.

19 North American Symptomatic Carotid Endarterectomy Trial Collaborators. The final results of the NASCET trial. *N Engl J Med* 1998; **339**:1415–25.

20 Chen ZM, Sandercock PAG, Pan HC, *et al.* Indications for early aspirin use in acute ischaemic stroke: a combined analysis of 40,000 randomised patients from the Chinese Acute Stroke Trial and the International Stroke Trial. *Stroke* 2000;**31**:1240–9.

21 Wardlaw JM, Del Zoppo G, Yamaguchi T. Thrombolysis for acute ischaemic stroke. In: Cochrane Collaboration. *Cochrane Library*. Issue 2. Oxford: Update Software, 2001.

22 Lindley Rl, Warlow CP. Why, and how, should trials be conducted? In: Zeman A, Emanuel L, eds. *Ethical dilemmas in neurology*. London: Saunders, 2000:73–86.

23 Chalmers I. Minimizing harm and maximising benefit during innovation in health care: controlled or uncontrolled experimentation? *Birth* 1986;**13**:155–64.

24 Freed CR, Greene PE, Breeze RE, *et al.* Transplantation of embryonic dopamine neurons for severe Parkinson's disease. *N Engl J Med* 2001; **344**:710–19.

25 Collins R, Doll R, Peto R. Ethics of clinical trials. In: Williams CJ, ed. *Introducing new treatments for cancer: practical, ethical and legal problems.* Chichester: John Wiley & Sons Ltd, 1992:49–65.

26 Rose G, Colwell L. Randomised controlled trial of anti-smoking advice: final (20 year) results. *J Epidemiol Community Health* 1992; **46**:75–7.

27 Moher D, Schulz KF, Altman DG, for the CONSORT Group. The CONSORT statement: revised recommendations for improving the quality of reports of parallel-group randomised trials. *Lancet* 2001; **357**:1191–4.

2 Why we need randomised controlled trials

TREVOR SHELDON AND ANN OAKLEY

One important context for health care research is the financial one: all health care is essentially a form of "legalised robbery". Money is extracted from households and given to health care providers, health care professionals, manufacturers, pharmaceutical companies, and so forth, and even possibly researchers who carry out the research. Governments, health insurance funds, businesses, and managed care networks are all very good at hiding the fact that health care is still extraction of money from households and its transfer to providers. This is an accounting identity: it must be so. But it does not mean that the amount of money spent on health care is equal to *investment* in health and welfare, because of course it depends on what happens to the money which is extracted from households to pay for health care. Is the money spent wisely on effective and appropriate approaches to promoting personal and public health, or is it wasted on ineffective, harmful, and/or unnecessarily expensive interventions? There are all sorts of devious ways in which providers can convince households that they should spend more and more of their income on health care. Much of the history of medicine is just such a confidence trick.[1] The implications are obvious: that we need to ensure spending is worthwhile; that it generates sufficient benefits; and that the distribution of those benefits is fair. Underneath it all it is quite important to remember the fundamental ethical principle, it is the public's money that is being spent in one way or another, and, therefore, the onus is on us to spend it wisely.

That is why we need evaluations. We need evaluations because it is not self evident that all health care spending is worthwhile in improving health or preventing ill health, on either a personal or societal level. Both biology and health care are tricky, highly complex systems and our understanding of how things work is still poor. We may have a good theory (for example, about a relevant biochemical mechanism, or about a set of economic relationships) as to why some form of spending should do us good, but these systems are so complex that accurately predicting the impact of what we do is extremely difficult. Often when we *think* we are doing good we are in fact doing harm, and that is why we need evaluation. There are logical reasons why health care providers should be over convinced, rather than under convinced, about the value of what they do: policies and interventions tend to be developed by enthusiasts, and this enthusiasm can be a source of bias. People believe in the value of what they are doing; the newest, latest thing is always particularly good, and, of course, governments always promote all their policies as good (even such absurdities as the Millennium Dome), since the essence of party politics is just this unevidenced conviction.

What we in the evaluation industry have to be interested in is accountability for what we do to the public, to the people who are funding health care in the first place. An evaluative culture is really important; it is not an optional extra. Policies are very often introduced without any evidence base, and that, in a sense, is fair enough, because we should not allow our lack of knowledge about how and whether something works to completely paralyse us. But what is worse is that, once such policies have been introduced, they are often not properly evaluated. One example is the whole quality initiative within the United Kingdom National Health Service: performance indicators; the performance assessment framework; clinical governance; and so on. These make up an extremely rich matrix of quality initiatives, but there is very little in the form of evaluation built into the matrix.[2] Or take the policy of merging hospitals, which was accompanied by many claims about savings and about improving outcomes, but very little in the way either of evidence or of sensible evaluations.[3] Fundholding and its abandonment are further examples of unevaluated policies.[4] Health Action Zones and Sure Start are current policy approaches to reducing health inequalities whose introduction has been followed by weak stabs at evaluation. When evaluation is an idea that occurs after the event, it is always difficult to carry out any kind of reliable evaluation. Policy makers and other experts are either certain that they *are* doing good and/or they are threatened by, or simply not interested in, gaining reliable knowledge about the effects of their actions.

The world is full of experts who want to spend our money and do things to us, who claim to know that it will improve our lives.

But *how* do they know? How do they know that what they do is actually making a difference, and making a positive difference? Randomised controlled trials have a critical role to play in delivering us from this chaos of well intentioned, but possibly misguided, expertise. The argument for randomised trials in health care evaluation is actually very simple, and exactly the same argument applies to other types of well intentioned intervention: the activities of social workers; criminal justice workers; teachers; psychotherapists; and so forth. There are three basic points. The first is that the counterfactual is rarely known. How do we know what would have happened if that particular intervention had not been introduced? Would the apparent improvement in outcome still be seen as due to the intervention, or might it, for example, be understood as "caused" by the curative effects of time, or perhaps by the general social support ("placebo") effects of research? Most trialists are, of course, well aware of the importance of having some kind of handle on the counterfactual. Designing and analysing trials makes one sharply aware of their advantages in facilitating baseline comparability (so that one is comparing outcomes in similar populations) and in controlling for regression to the mean, a point misunderstood by many people. Football is a good example. An average team, or quite a good team, has a run of bad luck. The response is not to wait for luck to change, but instead to change the manager. After the new manager comes in, the team draws with Manchester United, so it must be the manager, rather than regression to the mean, that made the difference. If you bring in a new manager when an average or a good team is doing badly, generally they are going to do better because you have intervened at a time that they were doing badly. Similarly, health care managers often come into trusts when things are going badly, so that their arrival, coinciding with improvement, is taken as proof of managerial efficiency. Only proper control comparisons can adequately deal with this problem of regression to the mean.

A second reason for using randomised trials to evaluate health care interventions is that most of these, whether clinical treatments, types of organisation, technologies, or policies, do, on the whole, have very modest effects.[5] There are very few interventions that have profoundly large effects where such trials are probably not necessary. It is because most have modest effects that you need a good comparison to try and reduce biases and confounding which could either mask or give the false impression of the existence of modest effect sizes. Thirdly, because you are dealing with complex systems, only the simplicity of trials can allow you to measure the effect of a change to that system. This is probably one of the most misunderstood aspects of trials. Social systems are highly complicated organisms; the fact that many things are changing all the time makes it very difficult to tell whether or not a single intervention, on its own, has been responsible for any change. Since it is virtually impossible to know about all the factors that may confound the attempt to establish the effects of an intervention when using an observational study, creating a control group is a simple method for dealing with that complexity. While anti-trialists often argue that trials are not appropriate because of social complexity,[6] it is precisely this aspect of the context in which research is done that gives this approach to evaluation the edge over any other.

There are many reviews comparing the results of quasi-experimental observational studies and randomised trials.[7,8] These often show differences in the direction of observational studies overestimating effects compared to randomised trials, though sometimes there is convergence; the problem is that we simply do not know what the conditions are under which you do get identical results.[9] Observational studies, particularly those that use routine data, have very poor information on context, on types of interventions, and the characteristics of people involved, so errors of interpretation are likely. There are a number of classic examples of misleading results derived from observational studies that have subsequently been shown in trials to have been biased. Three recent examples are hormone replacement therapy, dietary β-carotene, and school-based sex education.

Observational studies consistently showed a benefit of hormone replacement therapy in preventing coronary heart disease, but of course all sorts of selection bias are involved there, with the kinds of women taking hormone replacement being generally those with healthier lifestyles in the first place. A review of data from clinical trials of hormone replacement therapy showed no effect,[10] or even possibly an adverse effect.[11] Similarly, β-carotene was hailed in observational studies as beneficial, but a trial showed that, with some cancers like lung cancer among smokers, β-carotene supplementation may actually increase cancer incidence.[12] In these two examples there was a plausible scientific theory that giving women pre-menopausal levels of hormones would preserve the gender advantage for women in heart disease, and that supplementation of diet with one of the active health promoting constituents of fruit and vegetables would produce the health outcomes associated with a healthy diet. But, in each case, trials yielded different answers from observational studies and there was no evidence of the benefits claimed. A third example concerns the contentious area of sex education. Observational studies, compared to randomised trials, show exaggerated positive effects of sex education on the incidence of unintended teenage pregnancy.[13]

Well intentioned interventions can do harm as well as good. One of the most famous examples of this in the social care domain is the Cambridge Somerville Youth Study, a controlled trial carried out in the United States in the 1930s. It was an attempt to prevent delinquency through the intervention of "sustained friendly counselling". Seven hundred and fifty 10 year old boys were divided into two groups, and one group got an intervention from counsellors with social work training lasting on average five years. Data collected after five years showed more delinquency in the intervention group.[14] This picture of worse outcomes was maintained in subsequent follow ups in 1946, 1955, and 1975, when significantly more of the intervention group than the control groups had experienced "undesirable" outcomes, including criminal conviction, death before 35, alcoholism, schizophrenia, and manic depression.[15] It was noted at the time that, without a control group, the fact that two thirds of the boys avoided delinquency would have been interpreted as evidence of the success of the intervention.

Social workers are just as unhappy as many health care providers at such news about the unanticipated hazards of their favourite therapies. Fortunately, there is also good news. A nice contrast with the Cambridge Somerville Youth Study is the evidence about the effects of out of home daycare for preschool children, widely hailed by the authors of observational studies as spelling bad news for children's cognitive and social development, but shown in a number of randomised trials to have beneficial effects.[16] The most famous of these, the Perry Preschool Project, initiated in the early 1960s, has a follow up to date of 27 years. Results include early improvements in cognitive ability scores for the experimental group that "washed out" within a few years, but at age 15 there were significant differences in educational achievement and delinquency favouring the experimental group. Later follow up confirmed a pattern of higher education and employment rates, fewer unintended pregnancies, and less criminality among "programme graduates".[17,18]

There is a considerable history of trials being used successfully to evaluate social policy interventions,[19–22] thereby providing reliable evidence for policy makers to consider when making policy decisions. In the above examples, for instance, the evidence would suggest that for preventing criminal behaviour in young people, providing good quality daycare for preschool children is a better option than intensive social work services. Other policy interventions which have been evaluated in randomised trials include income maintenance[23] and housing allowance programmes,[24] labour force participation initiatives,[25] rehabilitation schemes for released prisoners,[26] and "contracting out" teaching in state schools to private firms to raise educational performance.[27]

Experimental research designs have come in for a lot of criticism within the social sciences, where some people see them as tools of a reductionist, positivist science with an intrinsic inability to capture the really important knowledge derived from personal observation.[28] Such positions are often embedded within a general postmodernist stance, which says that all knowledge is relative and there is no such thing as a hierarchy of evidence. The problem with these epistemological critiques is that they fail to provide any alternative method for minimising bias, and they fail to acknowledge that there *is* a real world in which people may be either helped or hindered by a whole range of medical, social, and educational interventions. The problem of being as sure as we can that what we say about the effectiveness of different approaches to promoting people's wellbeing is as reliable as possible exists right across the sciences. There is a lot of debate about the balance between theory and observation. In some of the social sciences theory is preeminent because theory makes careers; having a good theory, whether or not it makes empirical sense, gets you published.

The move against trials has created a new fashion for what is called "realistic" evaluation. This emphasises the need for a theory-led approach and gives more prominence to the importance of the contexts in which research is done, and the nature of the relationships between interventions and outcomes.[29] The argument is that the very complexity of social systems demands that we do not attempt to simplify and identify what works. On the contrary, the argument goes, this approach is doomed to failure; any conclusions we draw will be mechanistic at best and spurious at worst, because we will not have grasped what lies within the "black box" of the transformative process.

Of course many trials are poorly designed: they are over simplistic; have poor external validity; and largely ignore the interactions between outcomes, individuals, interventions, and context. But these are methodological challenges, not fundamental critiques.

Unfortunately, the retreat from experimentation seems to be accelerating in health care. One example is in the quality field, which is important because there is a huge amount of investment at the moment in quality improvement and quality initiatives. Don Berwick, an international guru on improving health care quality, who is in the Secretary of State for Health's advisory group said: "The rooting of health care in scientific research has generated some myopia about the preconditions for inference. When we try to improve a system we do not need perfect inference about a pre-existing hypothesis: we do not need randomisation, power calculations, and large samples."[30]

That is worrying, particularly given the results from studies of continuous quality improvement (CQI) which follow the same pattern found in the classic study by Sacks et al.,[31] which compared medical therapies that had been evaluated without controls, without concurrent controls, and then later with concurrent controls. There was a huge reduction in the percentage of interventions which showed benefit (from 79% to 20%): the better the control, the more conservative is the estimate of benefit.

The majority of continuous quality improvement studies are just before or after studies with no controls, and a vast majority of those show some improvement. The three randomised trials of continuous quality improvement show no impact.[32] Greineder et al.,[33] retracting the results of their earlier paper, explained how, when evaluating a continuous quality improvement intervention, the estimate of benefit was halved when moving from a simple before–after study to adding a comparison group: it was not a randomised trial, but at least it had a control. Continuous quality improvement, and similar interventions, can be evaluated using experimental approaches, and quality improvement will only mature when this becomes routine.[34] Continuous quality improvement and business process re-engineering take up a lot of resources in the National Health Service and dominate the minds of managers. So if their benefits are not that substantial, and managers are concerning themselves with things where there is little good evidence of effectiveness, we really do need to be worried.

Randomised trials are useful for evaluating health technologies, but we need to look at health service interventions as well. For example, we need rigorous evaluations of financing: how we rob households; how we pay health care practitioners; user charges; the configuration of hospitals; team work; regulation and quality control; performance management; and the use of performance indicators. There are no evaluations of performance indicators in the United Kingdom, but this does not prevent the approach being rolled out. Issues about skill mix and training are other candidates for proper evaluation: there is a whole area here which does potentially profoundly affect the efficiency or quality of care and the social distribution of these benefits.

There is, however, no magic about trials. An evaluation is not good just *because* it is a randomised trial. Many trials are poorly designed and executed, and these may well be worse than good observational studies. It is not hard to find trials, for example, which are uninformed by any theory; and very few are structured so as to find out about the processes involved in developing and implementing interventions. Why did an intervention only work for some people? What did its participants think of it? Why did only some people get it? Did everyone experience the same intervention? Insufficient numbers of trials combine quantitative data with qualitative data on people's experiences. Large, simple trials are a good idea, but we do need to try to understand things as well.[35] Unless we do this, it is difficult to interpret the results of some of these studies and impossible to know whether we can generalise from them. It worked there, but how can I take what was there and implement it here? What was it that was being evaluated? These questions are easier to answer with a drug than for models of care. We also need more involvement of research participants and obviously we need to increase generalisability. In short, there is a major methodological agenda ahead of us.

Trials can be done well, and they can be done in complex settings. For example, the Hutchinson Smoking Prevention Trial, which should be reporting soon, is a study of smoking prevention in schoolchildren, which we know is always a very difficult area in which to do evaluations. The trial randomised 40 school districts, included 8000 children, two consecutive cohorts and a 15 year follow up looking at knowledge, attitudes and behaviour both in school and beyond, firmly based on a reasonable theory: the social influences model. The researchers in the trial have achieved something like 99% teacher involvement, 86% fidelity to implementation, and 94% of the children have outcomes measured.[36] Similar ambitious designs have been achieved in two ongoing trials of peer led sex education in English secondary schools and social support for disadvantaged families. In the sex education trial 28 schools agreed to be randomised either to implement a short programme of sex education delivered by trained 15–16 year olds to 13–14 year olds in two successive cohorts or to carry on with their normal sex education. A six-year follow up is planned of the young people recruited to the trial, and outcomes include knowledge, attitudes, sexual behaviour, contraceptive use, unintended pregnancies, and sexually transmitted diseases. An important feature of the trial is the collection of qualitative process data, including through focus groups with young people, teacher interviews, and classroom observations.[37] In the social support trial, 731 new mothers in a disadvantaged urban area agreed to be randomised to either a supportive health visiting programme, community group support, or normal services. They also agreed to provide data through questionnaires and interviews on outcomes, including mothers' and children's health and health service use, maternal smoking, employment, and family wellbeing. A particular feature of this trial is the inclusion of many non-English speakers, and the use of interpreters both to recruit and to provide the interventions.[38]

Our two final observations concern clinical trials and social experimentation. Firstly, we know that routine care is a lottery: what you get often depends on who you see and where you go. There is no informed consent for this, and most people do not even realise that health care *is* part of a lottery. Furthermore, this state of affairs does not add to knowledge, because no one is making the comparisons. So perhaps we should just randomise instead, thereby turning the United Kingdom National Health Service into a laboratory and incorporating randomised trials into its fabric. Controlled random allocation would be part of the social contract; anyone coming to the National Health Service for treatment might be entered into a trial, so no specific informed consent would be needed for recruitment to any particular study. This is a difficult issue ethically, but stronger ethics and scientific control of what trials could be conducted within the United Kingdom National Health Service are both needed anyway.

Secondly, in terms of health and social policy, there is currently hardly any large scale social experimentation in Britain. We should try to persuade social and health policy makers to start to randomise more, to generate reliable evidence about the effectiveness of a whole range of policies. There are particularly strong arguments for randomisation as a method of resource allocation when resources are scarce, which they usually are in the public policy field.[38] A good example of how this can be done is in the recent evaluation of school breakfast clubs, carried out at the University of East Anglia. Randomisation should be the norm, rather than the esoteric exception. We need more formalised experimental approaches to knowledge, because this is a powerful way to improve the knowledge base for effective public policy. This model of continuous experimentation under strong scientific and public control is a democratic way of generating knowledge. It opens the research and evaluation process to public scrutiny at the same time as ensuring that those who intervene as practitioners and policy makers in other people's lives do so with the most benefit and the least harm.

References

1 McKeown T. *The role of medicine: dream, mirage or nemesis.* Princeton: Princeton University Press, 1979.
2 Sheldon TA, Maynard A, Watt I. Promoting quality in the NHS. *Health Policy Matters* 2001;**Issue 4, May**:1–4.
3 Ferguson B, Sheldon TA, Posnett J, eds. *Concentration and choice in health care.* London: Royal Society of Medicine Press Ltd, 1977.
4 Davies HTO, Nutley SM. The rise and rise of evidence in health care. *Public Money Manage* 1999;**19**:9–16.
5 Peto R, Collins R, Gray R. Large-scale randomized evidence: large, simple trials and overviews of trials. *Ann New York Acad Sci* 1993;**703**: 314–40.
6 Hunter D. Let's hear it for R & D. *Health Serv J* 1993;**15**:17.
7 Wright ME, Dixon MC. Community prevention and treatment of juvenile delinquency. *J Res Crime Delinq* 1977;**35**:67.
8 MacLehouse RR, Reeves BC, Harvey IM, Sheldon TA, Russell IT, Black AMS. A systematic review of comparisons of effect sizes derived from randomised and non-randomised studies. *Health Technol Assess* 2000;4(34):1–154.
9 Kunz R, Oxman A. The unpredictability paradox: review of empirical comparisons of randomised and non-randomised clinical trials. *BMJ* 1998;**317**:1185–90.
10 Hemminki E, McPherson K. Impact of postmenopausal hormone therapy on cardiovascular events and cancer – pooled data from clinical trials. *BMJ* 1997;**315**:149–53.
11 Josephson D. Women with heart disease cautioned about HRT. *BMJ* 1999;**318**:753.
12 Omenn GS, Goodman MD, Thornquist MD *et al.* Effects of a combination of beta carotene and vitamin A on lung cancer and cardiovascular disease. *N Engl J Med* 1996;**334**:1150–5.
13 Guyatt GH, DiCenso A, Farewell V, Willan A, Griffith L. Randomized trials versus observational studies in adolescent pregnancy prevention. *J Clin Epidemiol* 2000;**53**:167–74.

14 Powers E, Witmer H. *An experiment in the prevention of juvenile delinquency: the Cambridge-Somerville Youth Study.* New York: Columbia University Press, 1951.

15 McCord J. Consideration of some effects of a counselling program. In: Martin SE, Sechrest LB, Redner R, eds. *New Directions in the Rehabilitation of Criminal Offenders.* Washington, DC: National Academy Press, 1981.

16 Zoritch B, Oakley A, Roberts I. The health and welfare effects of daycare: a systematic review of randomised controlled trials. *Soc Sci Med* 1998;47:317–27.

17 Berrueta-Clement JR, Schwinhart LJ, Barnett WS, Epstein AS, Weikart DP. *Changed lives: the effects of the Perry Preschool Program through age 19.* Ypsilanti, MI: High/Scope Press, 1984.

18 Schweinhart LJ, Barnes HV, Weikart DP. *Significant benefits: the High/Scope Perry Preschool Study through age 27.* Ypsilanti, MI: High/Scope Press, 1993.

19 Boruch RF. *Randomized experiments for planning and evaluation.* Thousand Oaks, CA: Sage Publications, 1997.

20 Ferber R, Hirsch WZ. *Social experimentation and economic policy.* Cambridge: Cambridge University Press, 1982.

21 Oakley A. Public policy experimentation: lessons from America. *Policy Stud* 1998;19(2):93–114.

22 Oakley A. *Experiments in knowing: gender and method in the social sciences.* Cambridge: Polity Press, 2000.

23 Pechman JA, Timpane PM, eds. *Work incentives and income guarantees: the New Jersey Negative Income Tax Experiment.* Washington, DC: The Brookings Institution, 1975.

24 Friedman J, Weinberg DH, eds. *The great housing experiment.* Beverly Hills: Sage, 1983.

25 Manpower Development Research Corporation. *Summary and findings of the national supported work demonstration.* Cambridge, MA: Ballinger, 1980.

26 Rossi PH, Berk RA, Leniham KJ. *Money, work and crime: experimental evidence.* New York: Academic Press, 1980.

27 Gramlich EM, Koshel PP. Is real-world experimentation possible? The case of Educational Performance Contracting. In: Williams W, Elmore RF, eds. *Social Program Implementation.* New York: Academic Press, 1975.

28 Davies H, Nutley S, Tilley N. Debates on the role of experimentation. In: Davies HTO, Nutley SM, Smith PC, eds. *What works? Evidence-based policy and practice in public services.* Bristol: Policy Press, 2000.

29 Pawson R, Tilley N. *Realistic evaluation.* London: Sage Publications, 1997.

30 Berwick DM. A primer on leading the improvement of systems. *BMJ* 1996;312:619–622.

31 Sacks H, Chalmers TC, Smith H. Randomized versus historical controls for clinical trials. *Am J Med* 1982;**72**:233–40.
32 Shortell SM, Bennett CL, Byck GR. Assessing the impact of continuous quality improvement on clinical practice: what it will take to accelerate progress. *Milbank Quarterly* 1998;**76**:593–624.
33 Greineder DK, Loane KC, Parks P. Outcomes for control patients referred to a paediatric asthma outreach program: an example of the Hawthorne effect. *Am J Managed Care* 1998;**4**:196–202.
34 Goldberg HI. Continuous quality improvement and controlled trials are not mutually exclusive. *Health Serv Res* 2000;**35**:701–5.
35 Sheldon TA. It ain't what you do but the way that you do it. *J Health Serv Res Policy* 2000;**6**:3–5.
36 Mann SL, Peterson AV Jr, Marek PM, Kealey KA. The Hutchinson smoking prevention project trial: Design and baseline characteristics. *Prev Med* 2000;**30**:485–95.
37 Strange V, Forrest S, Oakley A (in press). A listening trial: qualitative methods within experimental research. In: Oliver S, Peersman G, eds. *Research matters in health promotion*. Buckingham: Open University Press.
38 Toroyan T, Roberts I, Oakley A. Randomisation and resource allocation: a missed opportunity for evaluating health care and social interventions. *J Med Ethics* 2000;**26**:319–22.

3 The importance of The *Cochrane Controlled Trials Register* to people doing and interpreting randomised trials

MIKE CLARKE

The Cochrane Controlled Trials Register was described in 1998 as the best single source of published trials for inclusion in systematic reviews.[1] This chapter shows why such a statement is justified, discusses how the register was compiled, and describes its importance to people who are designing a randomised trial or interpreting its results.

The need for a register of randomised trials

The lack of a comprehensive central repository of information on reports of randomised trials was recognised as one of the major challenges facing people who wanted to do systematic reviews when the Cochrane Collaboration was formed in 1993.[2] At that time, less than 20 000 reports of randomised trials could be readily identified in MEDLINE. This database contained many times that number of reports of randomised trials, but these could not be retrieved using simple, precise search strategies.[3] The Cochrane Collaboration has worked with the United States National Library of Medicine (which produces MEDLINE) to improve this over the subsequent years. The Collaboration has provided the information necessary to retag nearly 100 000 records in MEDLINE so that searchers of that database can now readily identify these as reports of trials.[4]

Records for these reports are also available within *The Cochrane Controlled Trials Register*, along with information from many other primary sources (including EMBASE, health care journals not indexed in MEDLINE, and conference proceedings) covering a wide range of areas of health care and interventions. *The Cochrane Controlled Trials Register* is updated and published quarterly as part of *The Cochrane Library*, which is available on CD ROM and the internet.[5] The focus of *The Cochrane Controlled Trials Register* is on reports of studies that might be eligible for inclusion in Cochrane reviews. This typically means reports of randomised trials. In addition, because its purpose is primarily to facilitate the conduct of systematic reviews, rather than to serve as a pristine register of randomised trials, it does contain some mistakes and some duplicates. However, as the first port of call for someone wishing to identify randomised trials, it is unequalled. The most recent release of *The Cochrane Controlled Trials Register* – in issue 4, 2001 of *The Cochrane Library* (October 2001) – contains records for more than 300 000 reports.

The fundamental rationale behind the need for a repository of information on randomised trials is that although many researchers hope that their randomised trials will prove influential in health care beyond their own locale, the means of disseminating their results can make it extremely difficult for this to happen. Every year, millions of articles about health care are published in tens of thousands of journals. For an individual to keep track of this literature, or even the subset that relates to their areas of interest, is clearly impossible. And yet, if someone wants to find good evidence of the effects of a particular intervention they need some way to find the relevant randomised trials or, ideally, a systematic review of these. With the growth of the Cochrane Collaboration, there are now more than 1000 Cochrane systematic reviews available in full text in *The Cochrane Library* but there are still many issues that have not been addressed by a Cochrane Review. People interested in these areas need to find the raw material – the randomised trials.

The compilation of *The Cochrane Controlled Trials Register*

This is where *The Cochrane Controlled Trials Register* represents such a valuable resource. It has been compiled through the searching of databases such as MEDLINE and EMBASE, the manual checking of hundreds of health care journals and conference proceedings and the preparation of records for ongoing or unpublished trials.

MEDLINE and EMBASE

MEDLINE and EMBASE are computerised bibliographic databases containing indexed records for articles published in the health care literature. They each contain millions of articles and can be searched to identify reports of interest. As noted above, before the establishment of the Cochrane Collaboration, MEDLINE contained less than 20 000 records that could be readily identified as reports of randomised trials. These were those that had been indexed with the Publication Type term "Randomised Controlled Trial". However, this term was only introduced in 1991 and, given that MEDLINE contains records going back as far as 1966, it could not have been assigned to a vast number of the records within the database that were reports of randomised trials. To help address this, through work done at the United Kingdom Cochrane Centre and the New England Cochrane Center, Providence Office (formerly the Baltimore Cochrane Center), 250 000 MEDLINE records have been retrieved using a specially designed search strategy.[3] The titles and abstracts of all these were read. Details of the 70 000 records that were judged to be definitely, or possibly, reports of randomised trials or quasi-randomised trials (that is, trials in which the allocation sequence is predictable such as alternation or date of birth) were passed to the United States National Library of Medicine. These have been retagged with the appropriate Publication Types in MEDLINE and can now be considered to be readily identifiable in that database. These records, along with those that have been identified as definite, or possible, randomised and quasi-randomised trials, are also included in *The Cochrane Controlled Trials Register*.

The UK Cochrane Centre has conducted a similar project for the EMBASE database. The titles and abstracts of approximately 100 000 records have been read and, from these, 33 000 reports of definite or possible randomised or quasi-randomised trials have been identified and included in *The Cochrane Controlled Trials Register*.[4]

Health care journals

Unfortunately, even though it is now easier to find reports of randomised trials that are in bibliographic databases such as

MEDLINE and EMBASE, there are still many reports that are not readily identifiable. These databases, and the handful of others that have been searched for *The Cochrane Controlled Trials Register*,[4] do not index all health care journals and even those that they do index might not be indexed in their entirety. Mistakes also happen and records that are in the databases might have been indexed incorrectly or with insufficient detail to be retrieved.

To address this, the Cochrane Collaboration has embarked on a worldwide effort to go through health care journals looking for reports of randomised trials (called "hand searching"). This has probably involved at least several dozen person-years of activity in the last eight years. This is one of the most collaborative aspects of the work within the Cochrane Collaboration. The people searching the journals do not simply look for reports of randomised trials of interest to them or their close colleagues. They check each article in every issue of the journals being searched to determine whether or not it is definitely or possibly a report of a randomised trial or a quasi-randomised trial, in any area of health and of any type of health care intervention. As of April 2001, more than 1700 journals have been, or are currently being, searched within the Cochrane Collaboration. Records are created for all reports identified in this way and these are submitted by the Cochrane Collaborative Review Groups and other Cochrane entities involved in this type of searching for inclusion in *The Cochrane Controlled Trials Register*.

Empirical work has been done to assess the yield of this type of searching for reports of randomised trials. A Cochrane Review of Methodology is ongoing to bring together comparisons of hand searching versus electronic searching.[6] One such project assessed the relative yield for 22 specialised health care journals published in the United Kingdom – all of which were, at least in part, indexed in MEDLINE. The reports of randomised trials found by the hand searching of three separate years for each journal (during the period 1970–1988) were compared with the retrieval from a simple MEDLINE search for the same journal years. A total of 714 reports of randomised trials were found by using a combination of the two types of search. Of these, 369 (52%) were identified only by hand searching and 32 (4%) were identified only by MEDLINE. Of those trials identified only by hand searching, 252 (68%) were meeting abstracts or published in supplements which MEDLINE had not indexed. Of the 462 randomised trials which had a MEDLINE record 117 (25%) were missed by the electronic search because they were not tagged with the relevant Publication Type terms.[7]

Conference proceedings

The above empirical study clearly shows that a large proportion of all reports of randomised trials might appear as meeting abstracts. This might not be too much of a problem for those interested in identifying reports of randomised trials if all of these studies reported at conferences went on to be reported in full, in health care journals. Unfortunately, this is not the case. Approximately half of the medical research presented at conferences and appearing as a printed abstract in the proceedings of the conference does not subsequently appear as a full article in a journal. Importantly, there are systematic differences between the half that do get published in full and the half that do not. The ones that are published in full tend to have more significant results.[8] Thus, a reviewer who fails to find relevant studies that were only ever published as meeting abstracts is likely to have found a biased set of studies, which might lead them to draw misleading or incorrect conclusions.

Several Cochrane Collaborative Review Groups are engaged in the searching of conference proceedings for randomised trials. Given the high yield of some of this searching and the evidence of bias relating to trials which will never appear in print elsewhere, this is a very important source of information for *The Cochrane Controlled Trials Register*. At the moment, the vast majority of the abstracts added in this way are not available from any other single source.

Unpublished trials

The above sources of records for *The Cochrane Controlled Trials Register* all rely on a report being published for the trial. However, a large proportion of randomised trials are never published, not even as a 250-word meeting abstract. The Medical Editors' Trials Amnesty was announced in 1997 as one attempt to address this. Editorials were published in approximately 100 health care journals, accompanied by a form to allow the submission of a very limited amount of information on any unpublished trials.[9] This has not been as successful as had been hoped. But, the information obtained on 150 unpublished trials is available in *The Cochrane Controlled Trials Register*.

A more successful approach to the identification of unpublished trials is the prospective registration of randomised trials at inception. *The Cochrane Controlled Trials Register* contains some records of this kind: notably, those submitted by Schering Healthcare Ltd (the United Kingdom division of the multinational drug company) for inclusion in 1997. However, the future of trial registration probably lies with online, internet-based systems, such as that being developed by Current Controlled Trials.

Why should trialists use *The Cochrane Controlled Trials Register*

There is increasing recognition that randomised trials of health care interventions should not be designed in isolation from what has gone before. Reviewing the trials that have already taken place, allows the person embarking on a new trial to learn from the experiences of the people who have done similar work in the past, in relation to the conduct of the trial. A systematic review of the existing evidence also allows them to ensure that the trial they are designing is the appropriate one to answer the questions that still need to be answered. *The Cochrane Controlled Trials Register* provides someone designing a trial with a single resource that will usually be the best starting point for a search for reports of randomised trials to review.

The need for a prior review has been recognised in the government document on Research Governance in England.[10] It is also accepted by funders, such as the Medical Research Council who require evidence of a systematic review in applications for clinical trials, and by ethics committees who use systematic reviews when assessing a proposal for a randomised trial.[11]

Having completed their trial, the trialists should ensure that they discuss it in the context of a systematic review of related studies.[12] Such a review allows the person reading the report of the new trial to assess what it adds to the existing research and to obtain an overall idea of the evidence on the issue. Without such a review, the readers will have to do their own review if they want the answers to these fundamental aspects of the interpretation of scientific research. Unfortunately, it has been shown that many trialists do not place their results in context appropriately.[13]

What can trialists do for *The Cochrane Controlled Trials Register*

Finally, besides getting involved directly in the work of the Cochrane Collaboration, everyone involved in a randomised trial should do whatever they can to ensure that others are aware of their work. After all, if they would like their trial to influence health care, they need people to be aware of it. When their trial is ongoing, trialists should ensure that it has been registered. When it has been completed, they should do what they can to get it published. And, when it has been published, they should send a reprint to the relevant Cochrane Collaborative Review Group.

Disclaimer

The views expressed in this chapter represent those of the author and are not necessarily the views or the official policy of the Cochrane Collaboration.

References

1 Egger M, Smith GD. Bias in location and selection of studies. *BMJ* 1998;**316**:61–6.
2 Chalmers I, Dickersin K, Chalmers TC. Getting to grips with Archie Cochrane's agenda. *BMJ* 1992;**305**:786–8.
3 Dickersin K, Scherer R, Lefebvre C. Identifying relevant studies for systematic reviews. *BMJ* 1994;**309**:1286–91.
4 Lefebvre C, Clarke MJ. Identifying randomised trials. In: Egger M, Altman DG, Davey Smith G, eds. *Systematic reviews in health care*. London: BMJ Publications, 2001:69–86.
5 The Cochrane Controlled Trials Register. In: Cochrane Collaboration. *Cochrane Library*. Issue 2. Oxford: Update Software, 2001.
6 Hopewell S, Clarke M, Lefebvre C, Scherer R. A comparison of hand searching with electronic searching to identify reports of randomised trials (Protocol for a Cochrane Methodology Review). In: Cochrane Collaboration. *Cochrane Library*. Issue 4. Oxford: Update Software, 2001.
7 Hopewell S, Clarke M, Lusher A, Westby M, Lefebvre C. A comparison of handsearching versus MEDLINE searching to identify reports of randomised controlled trials [Abstract]. *3rd Symposium on Systematic Reviews: Beyond the Basics*, July 2000 in Oxford.
8 Scherer RW, Langenberg P. Full publication of results initially presented in abstracts (Cochrane Methodology Review). In: Cochrane Collaboration. *Cochrane Library*. Issue 4. Oxford: Update Software, 2001.
9 Smith R, Roberts I. An amnesty for unpublished trials. *BMJ* 1997;**315**:622.
10 Research Governance in England. www.nhsetrent.gov.uk/trentrd/resgov/govhome.htm (accessed 11 Jul 2001).

11 Chalmers I. Using systematic reviews and registers of ongoing trials for scientific and ethical trial design, monitoring, and reporting. In: Egger M, Altman DG, Davey Smith G, eds. *Systematic reviews in health care*. London: BMJ Publications, 2001:429–43.
12 Begg C, Cho M, Eastwood S, *et al*. Improving the quality of reporting of randomised controlled trials. The CONSORT statement. *JAMA* 1996;**276**:637–9.
13 Clarke M, Chalmers I. Discussion sections in reports of controlled trials published in five general medical journals: islands in search of continents? *JAMA* 1998;**280**:280–2.

4 What have we learned from 50 years of randomised trials for people with schizophrenia?

CLIVE ADAMS

The advent of randomised controlled trials over fifty years ago coincided with a revolution in the care of people with schizophrenia. Drug treatments were being developed that would dramatically improve the mental state of those for whom little hope had previously existed. Psychiatrists welcomed the opportunity to test these drugs within randomised trials, strengthening their tradition of evaluative research.

The recent creation of registers of randomised trials, such as that developed by the Cochrane Schizophrenia Group, affords an opportunity to survey the quality of evaluative research within a well defined sampling frame. There are now many examples of surveys of trials published within specified journals,[1-3] including the pilot study for the work presented here.[4] However, research into the quality and content of trials across a whole subspecialty of health care, rather than within a specific journal, is less common.[5-9] This chapter presents and discusses studies designed to describe the characteristics of trials involving people with schizophrenia.[10]

The Register of Trials maintained by the Cochrane Schizophrenia Group

The Cochrane Schizophrenia Group's Register of Trials contains reports of published and unpublished controlled clinical trials in which allocation of treatment is, or is implied to be, at random. These studies relate to the care of those with schizophrenia and similar illnesses. The methods for compiling and maintaining this register have been described elsewhere.[11] In summary, for this analysis, studies were identified by hand searching key journals from 1948 to 1997, inclusive. Relevant conference proceedings were also hand searched. In addition, we searched databases that were of proven value for mental health literature (Biological Abstracts 1982–96, CINAHL 1980–96, *The Cochrane Library* Issue 3, 1997, EMBASE 1980–96, LILACS 1980–96, PsycLit 1974–96, PSYNDEX 1980–95, MEDLINE 1966–96, and Sociofile 1985–96). A total of 30 000 electronic records were checked and 6000 full copies of articles were obtained. At the end of 1997, when this survey was undertaken, the register contained 3181 publications, which referred to approximately 2500 trials.

Methods for the survey

Supported by a grant from the Medical Research Council, Ben Thornley and I surveyed the first 2000 trials, which were reported in 2275 publications. We recorded the type and date of publication, country of origin, and language of each study, and used a measure of methodological quality based on each trial's description of randomisation, blinding, and withdrawal from treatment.[12] This measure could produce a maximum score of five, for which the report had to have given appropriate methods of generating random assignment, appropriate blinding of participants and raters, and details on those who withdrew from the trial before its conclusion. This particular measure was chosen for its validity,[12] ease of use, and because low scores (indicating poor quality of reporting) are associated with an increased estimate of benefit.[13] We also recorded the size of the study, treatment setting, participants, interventions, and outcomes. One person coded most of the reports, and a 10% sample was recoded to test and ensure reliability. Data were analysed with Microsoft Excel.

Results

Reliability of coding

There was over 90% agreement in all variables except the numbers completing the study (70%) and listing of outcome instruments; in about 10% of reports the principal rater failed to identify one of the scales, often among several used.

Frequency of studies

The numbers of trials relevant to schizophrenia are rising steadily over time, from about 20 per year in the 1950s and 1960s to an average of nearly 75 per year in the past decade.

Sources of trials

Most of the 2275 reports were fully published in journals (85%, n = 1940), while the remainder were presented at conferences (11%, n = 253) or published as letters, dissertations, books, chapters, or product monographs (4%, n = 82). Most trials were reported in general psychiatric journals. The *Lancet* and *British Medical Journal* publish a few more schizophrenia trials than the *Journal of the American Medical Association* or the *New England Journal of Medicine* (33, 21, 6, 2 respectively), but all these widely read journals were limited sources of trials on this most serious and costly illness.

Most (97%, n = 2214) reports were published in English and over half were from North America (54%, n = 238). Just over one third of schizophrenia trials are from Europe (37%, n = 849) and 8% (n = 188) from the rest of the world. Trial output from North America is increasing at a faster rate (0.9 extra trials per year) than that from Europe (0.7 extra per year) and the rest of the world (0.3 extra per year).

Trial size

The average number of trial participants was 65 (median 50), with no discernible change over time. Only 20 trials (1%) raised the issue of the statistical power of the study. For an outcome such as "clinically important improvement" (to show a 20% difference between groups) a two-arm study would have to involve 300 people (α = 0.05, power 85%). Only 3% (n = 60) of studies involved more than 300 participants; 50% of trials were less than 50 people.

Setting

Only 14% of the total sample of trials (n = 272) were clearly community based, although the proportion increased. Even in the 1990s, however, the proportion was still small (23%, n = 135/587).

Interventions

Treatments were classed as "drug", "psychotherapy" (any treatment based on talking), "physical treatment" (such as electroconvulsive therapy and psychosurgery), "policy or care packages" (for example, case management and team treatment), and "other". Overall, 86% of trials (n = 1725/2000) evaluated the effects of 437 different drugs. Haloperidol, an effective antipsychotic with marked adverse effects,[14] however, was an increasingly frequent "benchmark" comparator; comparison of almost any moderately effective antipsychotic with haloperidol will result in the oft-vaunted claim of equal clinical effectiveness with a more favourable adverse effect profile. Overall, the proportion of drug trials has declined somewhat over time, with studies of psychotherapy and policy or care packages increasing.

Duration of treatment

Schizophrenia is often a life long illness. Over half of the trials, however, lasted six weeks or less (54%, n = 1082), and fewer than one fifth of the trials allowed more than six months to evaluate the treatments (19%, n = 382).

Measurement of outcome

One quarter of the studies (n = 510) did not use rating scales to measure outcomes. The remaining 1490 trials, however, used 640 different instruments, 369 of which were used only once. Most trials used between one and five instruments, but greater numbers were common, with one trial reporting use of 17 different outcome scales.

In an additional investigation, the details of which are described elsewhere,[15] 300 trials were randomly selected from the Cochrane Schizophrenia Group's Register. All comparisons between treatment and control groups using rating scales were identified, the publication status of each scale determined, and claims of a significant treatment effect recorded. Trials were more likely to report that a treatment was superior to control when an unpublished scale was used to make the comparison (relative risk 1.4, 95% confidence interval 1.1 to 1.7). According to a "face value" definition of treatment superiority, treatment was superior to control in 45% (n = 205/456) of comparisons. The "face value" definition was that the treatment group had a significantly better outcome, at a 5% level of significance, as measured by the rating scale at end point. Of these "face value" statistically significant comparisons, 36% (95%

confidence interval 30 to 43%, n = 74) were based on data from unpublished scales. The "gold standard" definition of statistical superiority was that the treatment group had a significantly better outcome, at the 5% level, on the overall (summary) score from the rating scale at the end of the trial. According to this rigorous "gold standard" definition, treatment was superior to control in only 20% (n = 90/456) of comparisons. Of these "gold standard" statistically significant comparisons, 44% (95% confidence interval 34% to 55%, n = 40) were based on data from unpublished scales.

Loss to follow up

Modern drug trials had remarkably high attrition. For example, loss to follow up by about eight weeks for clozapine studies was 16%, for risperidone it was 30%, for olanzapine 42% and for quetiapine 58%.

Quality of reporting

On average, quality of reporting was poor. Only 4% of the trials clearly described the methods of allocation (n – 80). Explicit descriptions of blinding were adequate in only 22% (n = 440), while some description of treatment withdrawals was given in 42% (n = 840). One per cent of the trials achieved a maximum quality score of five (n = 20). Just under two thirds (n = 1280) scored two or less, which means that they barely, if at all, described any attempt to reduce the potential for introduction of bias at allocation or rating of outcome, placebo effects, or the fate of all participants. A score of three or more was predefined as "better quality". Just 33% (n = 354/1062) of North American trials achieved this, compared with 36% (n = 262/724) of European trials and 43% (n = 77/180) of those from the rest of the world ($\chi^2 = 9.23$, $P < 0.01$). We found little evidence that the quality of trial reporting improved with time. From 1950 to 1997 the mean quality score was consistently poor (under 2.5).

Discussion

Our sample is likely to be biased in some respects. Searching was largely, but not exclusively, in English, and our ability to code articles in other languages, limited. However, it is unlikely that there are enough undiscovered large, high quality trials published in other languages to substantially change the results of this survey.

The first 2000 trials on the Cochrane Schizophrenia Group's Register were a subsample of around 5000 currently identified. High availability of a report would have increased the chance of early entry on to the register, and therefore of inclusion in the survey. Smaller, more recent surveys that have sampled from the 5000 studies,[15-16] suggest that the original sample of 2000 remains representative of all trials currently identified on the Cochrane Schizophrenia Group's Register.

Possible contributing factors to the limited quality

Trials relevant to people with schizophrenia are difficult to conduct. The illness, affecting only one percent of people at some point in their lives, may lead to chaotic behaviour and disordered thinking, erosion of insight and, often, considerable mistrust of health care professionals. These factors, along with the relatively weak tradition of multicentre, multinational trials, may have promoted limited study size and duration. In addition, the pursuit of reliable outcome measurement spawns the use of an extraordinary number of rating scales, one third of which were unpublished at time of use, and therefore of doubtful validity. This endeavour probably reflects not only the researchers' will to objectively quantify, but also the lack of statistical power in small trials to produce more clinically relevant outcomes; it is often possible to achieve *statistical* significance on these measures of doubtful *clinical* relevance with small numbers. Underlining their clinical irrelevance, scales are rarely used in clinical practice. In any event, the low quality of reporting in these trials probably results in a consistent 30–40% overestimate of benefit,[13,17-19] although, hopefully, this mediocre reporting will change with wider adoption of the CONSORT recommendations.[20]

Increasing complexity of trial design must contribute, at least in part, to attrition far greater than would be seen in routine clinical care. As a result, between 30 and 60% of data on the effects of the novel antipsychotic drugs are based on untested assumptions about the fate of people once they left the study, often applied by researchers who are employed by those with substantial pecuniary interests in the results. Also, as complexity increases, so does the expense of carrying out randomised trials relevant to the care of people with schizophrenia. In the United States, public and private institutions are increasingly taking on the financial burden of supporting schizophrenia trials. Strict entry criteria to these trials, however, make the generalisability of results problematic, even within the United States of America,[21] and only 2 to 4% of the world's population of people with schizophrenia live in North America.

Conclusions

The findings of this survey are as bad, if not worse, as those for other disciplines of health care.[1-3,5-9,18-19] This particularly detailed survey highlights how, with notable exceptions, half a century of trial research has produced small studies of limited quality, duration, and clinical utility. As the numbers of trials relevant to schizophrenia rise, the need for up to date systematic reviews of these studies increases. High quality systematic reviews can, however, never fully compensate for limited, poorly designed, conducted, or reported studies.

Inevitably the next 50 years will see many more similar studies, but there are now calls for well designed, well conducted, and properly reported clinically relevant randomised trials.[22,23] Future years should see more clinicians randomising people with schizophrenia into more studies that compare routine packages of care (around which there is genuine uncertainty as regards effectiveness and efficiency) and that measure outcomes of interest to clinicians, to policy makers, and to people with schizophrenia and their families.

References

1 Fahey T, Hyde C, Milne R, Thorogood M. The type and quality of randomised controlled trials (RCTs) published in United Kingdom public health journals. *J Public Health Med* 1995;**17**:469–74.
2 Lent V, Langenbach A. A retrospective quality analysis of 102 randomised trials in four leading urological journals from 1984–1989. *Urol Res* 1996;**24**:119–22.
3 Silagy CA. Developing a register of randomised controlled trials in primary care. *BMJ* 1993;**306**:897–900.
4 Ahmed I, Soares KVS, Seifas R, Adams CE. Randomised controlled trials in *Archives of General Psychiatry* (1959–1995): a prevalence study. *Arch Gen Psychiatry* 1998;**55**:754–5.
5 Chalmers I. A register of controlled trials in perinatal medicine. *WHO Chron* 1986;**40**:61–5.

6 Chalmers I, Hetherington J, Newdick M *et al*. The Oxford Database of Perinatal Trials: developing a register of published reports of controlled trials. *Control Clin Trials* 1986;7:306–24.

7 Cheng K, Ashby D, O'Hea U, Smyth R. The epidemiology of randomised controlled trials in cystic fibrosis. *Isr J Med Sci* 1996; 32:S260.

8 Nicolucci A, Grilli R, Alexanian AA, Apolone G, Torri V, Liberati A. Quality, evolution, and clinical implications of randomised, controlled trials on the treatment of lung cancer. A lost opportunity for meta-analysis. *JAMA* 1989;262:2101–7.

9 Vandekerckhove P, O'Donovan PA, Lilford RJ, Harada TW. Infertility treatment: from cookery to science. The epidemiology of randomised controlled trials. *Br J Obstet Gynaecol* 1993;100:1005–36.

10 Thornley B, Adams CE. Content and quality of 2000 controlled trials in schizophrenia over 50 years. *BMJ* 1998;317:1181–4.

11 Adams CE, Duggan L, Roberts L, Wahlbeck K, White P. The Cochrane Schizophrenia Group. In: Cochrane Collaboration. *Cochrane Library*. Issue 2. Oxford: Update Software, 2001.

12 Jadad AR, Moore RA, Carroll D *et al*. Assessing the quality of reports of randomised clinical trials: is blinding necessary? *Control Clin Trials* 1996;17:1–12.

13 Moher D, Pham B, Jones A *et al*. Does quality of reports of randomised trials affect estimates of intervention efficacy reported in meta-analyses? *Lancet* 1998,352:609–13.

14 Joy C, Lawrie S, Adams CE. Haloperidol versus placebo for schizophrenia. *Cochrane Database Syst Rev* 2001;2:CD001087.

15 Marshall M, Lockwood A, Bradley C, Adams CE, Joy C, Fenton M. Unpublished rating scales: a major source of bias in randomised controlled trials of treatments for schizophrenia. *Br J Psychiatry* 2000;176:249–52.

16 Wahlbeck K, Adams C, Thornley B. Much to improve: a survey of controlled Nordic schizophrenia trials. *Nord J Psychiatry* 2000;54: 105–8.

17 Schulz KF, Chalmers I, Altman DG, Grimes DA, Dore CJ. The methodologic quality of randomisation as assessed from reports of trials in specialist and general medical journals. *Online J Curr Clin Trials* 1995; Doc No 197.

18 Gøtzsche P. Methodology and overt and hidden bias in reports of 196 double-blind trials of nonsteroidal antiinflammatory drugs in rheumatoid arthritis. *Control Clin Trials* 1989;10:31–56.

19 Chalmers TC, Celano P, Sacks HS, Smith Jr H. Bias in treatment assignment in controlled clinical trials. *N Engl J Med* 1983;309: 1358–61.

20 Begg C, Cho M, Eastwood S *et al*. Improving the quality of reporting of randomised controlled trials. The CONSORT statement. *JAMA* 1996,276:637–9.

21 Wells K. Treatment research at the crossroads: the scientific interface of clinical trials and effectiveness research. *Am J Psychiatry* 1999; **156**:5–10.

22 Hotopf M, Churchill R, Lewis G. Pragmatic randomised controlled trials in psychiatry. *Br J Psychiatry* 1999;**175**:217–23.

23 Roland M, Torgerson DJ. What are pragmatic trials? *BMJ* 1998; **316**:285.

5 Big is still beautiful: why we still need large simple trials

LELIA DULEY AND JOSÉ VILLAR

Randomised trials are now well accepted as the most valid means of evaluating medical or surgical treatments, screening, or preventive manoeuvres, as well as health, nutritional, social, and educational interventions.[1-3] The beauty of randomisation is that it is the only certain way of eliminating bias in how people are allocated to the intervention of interest. When comparing the outcome for groups of people exposed to different interventions it is possible during the analysis to control for known risk factors, but randomisation is the only way to control for any unknown factors that may influence outcome.

Although the use of randomised trials has increased dramatically in recent years, there remains great scope for wider application to important questions in health care. In many situations, if we want to find "truth" we need large trials. In this chapter we will argue that the need for large trials is greater than ever before, and, that to be affordable and feasible within a sensible timeframe, these trials must be simple.

Why do we continue to need large simple trials?

Powerful arguments have been put forward to support the need for large scale randomised trials.[4,5] In modern medicine, the best that can realistically be expected from most new treatments is a moderate effect. So we need to design studies that can discriminate reliably between differences in outcome that are moderate but still worthwhile, and differences that are too small to have any clinical value. These studies must guarantee strict control of bias, by proper randomisation (supported by sound design and appropriate

Why we still need large simple trials

- To reduce random errors until they are very small.

- To have the power to assess effects on rare outcomes.

- To have the power to assess effects in clinically important subgroups.

- To have the power to demonstrate clinical equivalence.

- To make it possible to do cluster randomisation trials.

- So that results are applicable to a wide range of people and settings.

statistical analysis), and strict control of the play of chance, which requires large numbers. To assess moderate benefits reliably, we must be sure that moderate biases and moderate random errors have been avoided.[4] This leads to the need for large numbers of properly randomised patients, with adequate numbers of events, which can be achieved by either large simple randomised trials and/or by systematic reviews of randomised trials.

For example, in the late 1980s a systematic review suggested that antiplatelets during pregnancy would more than halve the risk of pre-eclampsia,[6] and there were hopes for similar reductions in the more substantive outcomes of stillbirth or neonatal death, preterm birth and intrauterine growth restriction. The trials in this review were small. Subsequent trials, the largest of which recruited nearly 10 000 women,[7] failed to confirm these benefits. A recent systematic review, which identified 39 trials and over 30 000 women (eight of these trials recruited >1000 women), has now shown that antiplatelets reduce the risk of pre-eclampsia by 15% and the risk of stillbirth or neonatal death by 14%.[8] Not one of the individual studies was large enough to detect these moderate, but clinically important, benefits.

If the treatment effect is large, it is obvious without the need for randomised trials. Trials were not necessary when penicillin was first introduced, for example. However, for most interventions aimed at most of today's priority diseases, it is unrealistic to hope for such large effects on mortality or morbidity. Some treatments do have large effects on other less substantive outcomes, or on intermediate mechanisms of pathophysiology: drugs readily lower blood pressure, blood lipids and blood glucose; streptokinase can dissolve coronary thrombi; and tumour growth can be controlled temporarily by radiotherapy or chemotherapy. Although effects on these intermediate outcomes may initially appear to be large, effects on the more fundamental outcomes of mortality or severe morbidity are usually more modest. For example, it is suggested that women with mild to moderate pregnancy-induced hypertension should be treated with antihypertensive drugs. There is good evidence that these drugs reduce blood pressure, but a recent systematic review failed to confirm beneficial effects on other more substantive outcomes, such as perinatal death, preterm birth or intrauterine growth restriction.[9]

Large trials are essential for assessment of morbidity as well as mortality. Increasingly it is being accepted that they are also necessary for reliable assessment of major disability and other substantive measures of morbidity. Someone with multiple sclerosis, schizophrenia, or diabetes will want to know whether they will be able to continue their normal day to day activities, care for their children, and stay in work. Scans, scales, and serum levels are very interesting to researchers, and provide comfortable sample size estimates for trials, but have little relevance to people if they are not directly related to specific symptoms or how the person is likely to function. To provide the kind of information that is meaningful to users of the health services we need large scale unbiased evidence. It seems logical too that people will be more willing to participate in trials if they can see that the information being generated will be of direct relevance to them. Consulting with consumers of health care will help identify outcomes that are important and relevant to the people we aim to help, a benefit to all.[10]

Generating really large scale randomised evidence will reduce random errors and bias, until both are tiny. This allows reliable assessment of any real, but moderate, effects of the intervention. Random errors can be reduced more easily and cheaply by using large observational datasets, which in many instances are collected already. The problem with such datasets, however, is that the potential for big selection biases cannot be controlled, particularly for those variables for which data were not collected. It has been argued that observational data can give the same answers as randomised trials,[11,12] but if they do so it is likely to be by chance.[13] We cannot safely base decisions about treatment on observational studies when the best that can be expected from these treatments is moderate improvements in death or disability.

Reducing the potential for bias is equally important when evaluating complex health care interventions. For example, a large body of observational evidence, collected during the 1970s and 1980s, showed a strong inverse relationship between the number of antenatal care visits and the risk of having a low birthweight baby, or a perinatal death.[14] Subsequent large randomised trials in both developed and developing countries have failed to demonstrate any protective effect, on low birthweight or perinatal mortality, of antenatal care delivered with a large number of visits rather than with a reduced number of visits.[15]

Some advantages of large simple trials

Generating reliable and relevant evidence

"Simple" in the context of large trials is a misleading term. "Pragmatic" may be a more appropriate way of describing this type of study. These trials are difficult and challenging projects. To be successful they need enormous effort in the design and planning of every aspect of recruiting, treating, and assessing patients. This preparatory phase will often take several years. Nevertheless, it is well worthwhile, as the results of large trials such as these will provide a reliable basis for future worldwide clinical practice. The potential impact of large trials is already clear. For example, in cardiovascular disease,[16] stroke,[17] and perinatal care.[18] In Chapter 4 Clive Adams describes how trials for people with schizophrenia have used complex eligibility criteria, cumbersome trial procedures, and outcome measures that have little relevance to clinical practice. They have therefore been small, of relevance to only a narrow spectrum of patients, and have failed to follow up a high proportion of participants beyond the first few weeks. Simplifying schizophrenia trials offers the exciting prospect of generating the sort of large scale randomised evidence that could really make a difference to the lives of people with schizophrenia.

Trials in emergency situations

Trials in emergency situations are always difficult, but they become feasible if the eligibility criteria and procedure for trial entry are simple. For example, the Collaborative Eclampsia Trial demonstrated that it is possible to conduct trials to evaluate care for women with eclampsia.[19] In this trial the aim was to deliver care at least as fast, if not faster, than within the routine health services. This was achieved by using consecutively numbered sealed treatment packs for trial entry, and 1687 women were recruited. The treatment packs were so successful that many hospitals wanted to continue using them after recruitment to the trial closed.[20] "Eclampsia packs" have now become part of standard practice in many hospitals.

Enhanced collaboration

Simple trials make widespread collaboration more feasible. More complex studies often involve only those who work in sophisticated and well resourced research centres. Such places are rarely typical, or representative, of those with the greatest need. Simple, pragmatic trials make collaboration within non-academic institutions and low to middle income countries possible. This has many advantages. As well as evaluating interventions in a relevant setting, these large collaborative groups will facilitate dissemination and implementation of the results. Those who collaborate on trials are more likely to incorporate the results of these trials into their clinical practice.[21] Collaboration in developing countries has an important role both in generating evidence, and facilitating implementation.

Rare but serious conditions

Evaluation of interventions for rare but serious conditions, such as eclampsia or serious head injury, requires large sample sizes. These can only be obtained by extensive worldwide collaboration. As discussed above, such collaboration is only likely to be possible within simple pragmatic trials.

How to do large simple trials

To recruit really large numbers of people over a reasonable period of time, and at an affordable cost, large trials need to be simple and pragmatic (see Box). Complexity is a barrier to recruitment, interferes with clinical practice, encourages participants to leave the study early, and restricts generalisability of the results. If assessing eligibility is complex, or based on criteria not widely used in clinical practice, many eligible patients will not be randomised and the results will only apply to the relatively narrow group of patients recruited. For rapid recruitment of large numbers of people,

Some advantages of simple pragmatic trials

- Feasible to recruit really large numbers of people.
  - simple eligibility criteria
  - simple trial entry procedure

- Conducted within the existing health services.
  - intervention feasible without additional staff or technology
  - data collection based on what is likely to be available

- Considerably less expensive than more complex studies.

- Minimal additional work for already busy clinicians.

- Encourages participants to stay in the study.

- More complete and better quality data.

- Simpler data management.

- Results relevant to clinical practice in a wide range of settings.

eligibility criteria and the procedure for trial entry must be simple, so that they can be adapted and integrated into existing clinical practice. For example, screening for inclusion in the WHO Misoprostol Third Stage Trial,[22] which recruited over 18 000 women, included only four questions and there was no test or complex clinical examination. This trial recruited 65% of the screened women. The Collaborative Eclampsia Trial[19] recruited 1687 women, by far the largest trial on this topic. Although one factor in recruitment was the high prevalence of eclampsia in participating centres, equally important was that enrolling a woman in the trial made her clinical care easier than normal practice for the attending staff.

The intervention should be feasible to deliver within the existing health services. It should not require staff or technology unlikely to be available at the time of recruitment. Data collection must be simple and based on information likely to be readily available in routine clinical notes. It should not be time consuming or difficult to collect. Information should only be collected if it is specified within the protocol as part of the planned analyses, and this should all be clinically relevant. No effort is then wasted collecting information that is unlikely ever to be used, or that has little clinical relevance. For example, in large trials it is unnecessary to collect multiple baseline variables, because if randomisation was correctly conducted and the allocation adequately concealed, the groups will be well balanced at trial entry. Only data for important prognostic variables need therefore be collected. As has been said before,[4] usually it is of far greater value to collect 10 times less data on 10 times more patients.

Demonstrating equivalence

Increasingly, a range of alternative interventions are available for the same condition. New treatments are advocated with the claim of equal effectiveness, but fewer or less severe side effects, easier mode of administration, or better cost effectiveness than standard therapy. Demonstrating that the claim of clinical equivalence is justified often requires large sample sizes. To demonstrate that any difference between treatment effects is clinically unimportant will require a larger sample size than demonstrating a difference that is sufficiently large to be clinically important.[23]

The importance of demonstrating equivalence depends on the importance of the condition, and of the potential additional advantages of the alternative agents. For example, early antipsychotic drugs for treatment of schizophrenia dramatically improved prognosis, but at the cost of frequent unpleasant and debilitating side effects. Each new wave of drugs is claimed to have equal effectiveness as those early agents but with a better side effect profile. These newer drugs are also several hundred times more expensive than the older agents. If the new drugs are more acceptable to people with schizophrenia, however, they may be more willing to continue to take them regularly. This improved compliance may reduce relapse. To date, trials have not been large enough to either confirm or to refute the claim of equal effectiveness, and the overall cost effectiveness of the new drugs remains controversial.[24,25]

Cluster randomisation

There is a growing interest in the use of cluster randomisation or community trials. For most trials the basic unit of randomisation is the individual person being allocated to a specific intervention or to a control or placebo. Other units (clusters) of randomisation such as clinics, hospitals, physicians, or families can be used, and are particularly attractive for evaluation of health services.[26-28] Advantages of cluster randomisation trials[29] are that they reduce "contamination" of the interventions between groups, they can increase participation, and they allow for better administrative and logistic organisation in implementing the intervention.

A disadvantage of cluster trials is that they often need to be larger than a comparable trial based on individual randomisation. If there is high homogeneity within each cluster, such as families or medical practices, the number of clusters within the trial will need to be large. The unit for analysis should be the cluster, rather than individuals. If the unit of inference of the results is the individual rather than the original cluster, such an analysis can be conducted but an adjustment for the effect of clustering is needed, which requires a larger sample size for the same statistical power. Cluster randomised trials are usually less efficient than individually randomised trials, because the responses of individuals within a cluster tend to be more similar than responses of individuals in different clusters.

Global partnerships

Often, to recruit sufficiently large numbers of people requires international collaboration.[30] These international partnerships develop slowly, and are not without difficulties or cost. Developing a trial protocol with input from a diverse group of people requires searching for compromises with which everybody is comfortable, and that every centre is able and willing to follow. This may introduce methodological difficulties, however. For example, in the WHO Antenatal Care Trial,[31] which tested the hypothesis that a reduced number of antenatal visits is as good as the more usual higher number of visits, there was concern that too flexible a protocol might actually bring the two interventions closer to each other, as had been the case in previous trials.[15] Protocol flexibility needs to be a balance between allowing continuation of routine practices whilst maintaining methodological quality in trial procedures.

Efficient communication between the trial coordinating centre and individual hospitals is crucial in order to resolve any problems without delay, and may present considerable challenges. Consent for participation in trials raises further issues, particularly as different countries will have different procedures and accepted norms. Most of these difficulties can be overcome through regular consultation that is sensitive to local norms, values, and beliefs. Partnerships based on mutual trust and respect are essential for the success of large collaborative trials. There is a growing demand for evidence from high quality trials. International collaboration offers a feasible, enjoyable, and productive route for addressing clinical questions of global importance.

Although building these global partnerships is difficult and requires long term commitment, we believe the advantages, as discussed below, outweigh the difficulties.

Rapid recruitment

A growing number of trials across a wide range of specialties have now demonstrated that large scale international collaboration is feasible and productive, in both developed and developing countries. For example, the Term Breech Trial recruited over 2000 women from 22 countries,[32] the International Stroke Trial[17] recruited 20 000 patients from 36 countries and the Magpie Trial Collaborative Group[33] involves 33 countries across four continents. In these studies, extensive international collaboration was essential to achieve target recruitment within a reasonable timeframe.

Changing practice

Trials have little value if their results are not incorporated into clinical practice. In large collaborative trials, local or national dissemination of the results is often the responsibility of the local coordinator. This is particularly important when there are barriers to dissemination, such as language or poor access to the medical literature. Lack of access to up to date information is an important problem in developing countries. Participation in large international trials ensures that these hospitals and clinical units have immediate access to the results once the trial is completed. The local coordinator is also likely to present the trial results in national and regional meetings, and may publicise them in local journals. This will facilitate dissemination, and may help implementation as there is evidence that participation in a trial means you are more likely to incorporate the results into your clinical practice.[21]

Results from these international trials are relevant to a wide range of clinical settings. For example, even when a study is conducted only in developing countries, the results can be extrapolated to, and benefit patient care in, developed countries too. The Collaborative Eclampsia Trial[19] has changed practice in the United Kingdom.[34] A trial conducted in Kenya on treatment of otitis media in children has implications for clinical practice in both developing and developed countries.[35,36]

Research capacity building

"Global partnerships" is an appropriate term for this approach as collaborating in this way increases the knowledge and experience of coordinators and country investigators alike. Continuing involvement in international trials enhances essential research capacity and develops the skills of staff working at individual centres, as well as facilitating networking. Each person contributes different cultural, logistical and practical perspectives, and part of the challenge of developing the "esprit de corps", as discussed in Chapter 7, is to manage and channel this great potential in a mutually creative way.

Pilot studies

Another advantage of large scale collaboration is the possibility of conducting pilot studies, when required, before the main trial is initiated. Within any multicentre trial, different centres will be ready to start at different times, allowing selection of suitable sites to test the optimal dose or develop procedures. For example, a pilot trial to select the optimal misoprostol dose for the WHO Misoprostol Third Stage Trial[37] recruited 600 women in seven weeks at two of the nine centres that were subsequently part of the main trial.

An example of a large simple trial

The Collaborative Eclampsia Trial[19] illustrates many of the issues discussed in this chapter. Eclampsia, the occurrence of a convulsion superimposed on the syndrome of pre-eclampsia, is a rare but serious complication of pregnancy. An estimated 50 000 women die every year following an eclamptic convulsion, which is 10% of direct maternal deaths.[38] Much of the discussion on how to care for these women has centred on anticonvulsant use, and controversy about which drug to use raged throughout most of the 20th century. By the early 1990s the most widely used were magnesium sulphate, diazepam and phenytoin. There was huge geographic variation in practice: magnesium sulphate being standard practice in the US, but rarely used in the United Kingdom, where diazepam and phenytoin were preferred. Despite strong opinions about the choice of drug, there was little reliable evidence. A systematic review at that time identified four trials with a total of 76 women randomised.[39,40]

This was the background to the Collaborative Eclampsia Trial, which compared magnesium sulphate with diazepam and with phenytoin. The trial was pragmatic, a woman was eligible if she had a clinical diagnosis of eclampsia. This simple eligibility criterion reflected clinical practice, as any delay in initiating treatment would have been unethical as well as impractical. Women were recruited from 27 hospitals in nine countries in South America, Africa and India. They were entered into the trial by opening the next in a consecutively numbered series of treatment packs. Each pack had a label on the lid, which requested the woman's name, her blood pressure and whether or not she had delivered. Once this label was completed she was in the trial. Each pack was sealed with paper tape, tied with string, and the string was sealed with wax. The pack was easy to open, but could not be tampered with without breaking the seal. The aim was that women recruited to the trial should receive treatment faster than those not recruited.

Each treatment pack included sufficient allocated drug for treatment for the full 24 hours, along with everything required to give the first dose.[41] They were identical in size, weight and feel. The packs were always placed in the same place as the hospital supply of anticonvulsant drugs for women with eclampsia. Two or three boxes were left out at any one time, placed in consecutive order, the next pack always on top ready to be grabbed when needed. In one hospital, trial entries started arriving out of order; we discovered this was because the cleaner was dusting the boxes and putting them back in the wrong order. We suggested they be left to gather dust.

In total, 1687 women were recruited, double the expected sample size. Several hospitals liked the treatment packs so much they kept on randomising after the end of the study. Accrual was 97%, with only 55 eligible women not randomised. Overall 99% of women received the allocated treatments, with 99.6% follow up for primary outcomes. Just 2.7% of the packs were opened out of order, on enquiry the reasons were all human error rather than bias.

The results showed that women had fewer recurrent fits if they received magnesium sulphate rather than diazepam (relative risk 0.48, 95% confidence interval 0.36 to 0.63) or magnesium rather than phenytoin (relative risk 0.33, 95% confidence interval 0.21 to 0.53). This effect was consistent across both the prestated subgroups: whether the women had an anticonvulsant before trial entry; and whether they had delivered before trial entry. In the phenytoin comparison the comparative benefit was even stronger, with effects on some secondary outcomes also favouring magnesium sulphate. This trial has had considerable impact, but dissemination and implementation is still ongoing. Magnesium sulphate is now on the WHO list of essential drugs. Nevertheless it is still not available in some developing countries, particularly in Africa.[42] The Royal College of Obstetricians and Gynaecologists has also incorporated magnesium sulphate into its guidelines for practice. In the United Kingdom, magnesium sulphate has become the drug of choice for eclampsia.[34,43] This large, simple study, designed to address a question relevant to developing countries, has changed practice in a wide range of settings.

In conclusion, large trials are much needed to evaluate preventive strategies, treatments, and health services. They are particularly important if the condition is rare, the expected impact is moderate, equivalence is being tested, or the unit of randomisation is a cluster rather than individuals. Large trials require collaboration among many research groups, and this can be achieved in both developing and developed countries. All forms of care, whether drug or non-drug, should be properly evaluated before being introduced into clinical practice. Large, simple, pragmatic trials play a central role in this process.

References

1 Collins R, MacMahon S. Reliable assessment of the effects of treatment on mortality and major morbidity, I: Clinical trials. *Lancet* 2001; 357:373–80.
2 Stephenson J, Imrie J. Why do we need randomised controlled trials to assess behavioural interventions? *BMJ* 1998;316:611–13.

3 Villar J, Carroli G. Methodological issues of randomised controlled trials for the evaluation of reproductive health interventions. *Prev Med* 1996;**25**:365–75.

4 Collins R, Peto R, Gray R, Parish S. Large-scale randomised evidence: trials and overviews. In: Weatherall DJ, Ledingham JGG, Warrell DA, eds. *Oxford Textbook of Medicine Vol 1, 3rd ed*. Oxford: Oxford University Press, 1996:21–32.

5 Yusuf S, Collins R, Peto R. Why do we need some large simple randomised trials? *Stat Med* 1986;**3**:409–20.

6 Collins R. Antiplatelet agents for IUGR and pre-eclampsia. In: Chalmers I, ed. *Oxford Database of Perinatal Trials*. Version 1.2, disk issue 4. Oxford: Oxford University Press, 1990.

7 CLASP (Collaborative Low-dose Aspirin Study in Pregnancy) Collaborative Group. CLASP: a randomised trial of low-dose aspirin for the prevention and treatment of pre-eclampsia among 9364 women. *Lancet* 1992;**343**:619–29.

8 Duley L, Henderson-Smart D, Knight M, King J. Antiplatelet drugs for prevention of pre-eclampsia and its consequences: a systematic review. *BMJ* 2001;**322**:329–33.

9 Abalos E, Duley L, Steyn DW, Henderson-Smart DJ. Anti-hypertensive drug therapy for mild to moderate hypertension during pregnancy (Cochrane Review). In: Cochrane Collaboration. *Cochrane Library*. Issue 2. Oxford: Update Software, 2001.

10 Chalmers I. The perinatal research agenda: whose priorities? *Birth* 1983;**18**:137–41.

11 Concoto J, Shah N, Horwitz RI. Randomised controlled trials, observational studies, and the hierarchy of research designs. *N Engl J Med* 2000;**342**:1887–92.

12 Benson K, Hartz AJ. A comparison of observational studies and randomised controlled trials. *N Engl J Med* 2000;**342**:1878–86.

13 Elbourne D, Pocock S. Randomised trials or observational tribulations? *N Engl J Med* 2000;**342**:1907–9.

14 Quick J, Greenlick M, Rogmann K. Prenatal care and pregnancy outcome in an HMO and general population: a multivariate cohort analysis. *Am J Public Health* 1981;**71**:381–90.

15 Villar J, Khan-Neelofur D. Patterns of routine antenatal care for low-risk pregnancy (Cochrane Review). In: Cochrane Collaboration. *Cochrane Library*. Issue 2. Oxford: Update Software, 2001.

16 ISIS-4 (Fourth International Study of Infarct Survival) Collaborative Group. ISIS-4: a randomised factorial trial assessing early oral captopril, oral mononitrate, and intravenous magnesium sulphate in 58 050 patients with suspected acute myocardial infarction. *Lancet* 1995;**345**: 669–85.

17 International Stroke Trial Collaborative Group. The International Stroke Trial (IST): a randomised trial of aspirin, subcutaneous heparin,

both, or neither among 19 435 patients with acute ischaemic stroke. *Lancet* 1997;**349**:1569–81.

18 Enkin M, Keirse M, Crowther C, Duley L, Hodnett E, Hofmeyr GJ. *The Guide to Effective Care in Pregnancy and Childbirth*, 3rd ed. Oxford: Oxford University Press, 2000.

19 The Eclampsia Trial Collaborative Group. Which anticonvulsant for women with eclampsia? Evidence from the Collaborative Eclampsia Trial. *Lancet* 1995;**345**:1455–63.

20 Duley L, Mahomed K. Magnesium sulphate in eclampsia. *Lancet* 1998;**351**:1061–2.

21 Ketley D, Woods KL. Impact of clinical trials on clinical practice: example of thrombolysis for acute myocardial infarction. *Lancet* 1993; **342**:891–4.

22 Gülmezoglu AM, Villar J, Ngoc NN *et al.* for the WHO Collaborative Group to Evaluate Misoprostol in the Management of the Third Stage of Labour. The WHO multicentre double-blind randomised controlled trial to evaluate the use of misoprostol in the management of the third stage of labour. *Lancet* 2001 (in press).

23 Jones B, Jarvis P, Lewis JA, Effutt AF. Trials to assess equivalence: the importance of rigorous methods. *BMJ* 1996;**313**:3–4.

24 Geddes J, Freemantle N, Harrison P, Bebbington P. Atypical antipsychotics in the treatment of schizophrenia: systematic overview and meta-regression analysis. *BMJ* 2000;**321**:1371–6.

25 Prior C, Clements J, Rowett M. Users' experiences of treatments must be considered. *BMJ* 2001;**322**:924.

26 Piaggio G, Carroli G, Villar J *et al.* Methodological considerations on the design and analysis of an equivalence stratified cluster randomisation trial. *Stat Med* 2001;**20**:401–16.

27 Donner A, Khan N. *Design and analysis of cluster randomisation trials in health research.* London: Arnol Publishers Limited, 2000.

28 Donner A, Piaggio G, Villar J *et al.* Methodological considerations in the design of the WHO antenatal care randomised controlled trial. *Paediatr Perinat Epidemiol* 1998;**12**(suppl 2):59–74.

29 Donner A, Piaggio G, Villar J. Statistical methods for the metaanalysis of cluster randomisation trials. *Stat Med Res* 2001 (in press).

30 Gülmezoglu M, Villar J, Hofmer J, Duley L, Belizán JM. Randomised trials in perinatal medicine: global partnerships are the way forward. *Br J Obstet Gynaecol* 1998;**105**:1244–7.

31 Villar J, Ba'aqeel H, Piaggio G *et al.* for the WHO Antenatal Care Trial Research Group. WHO antenatal care randomised trial for the evaluation of model of routine antenatal care. *Lancet* 2001;**357**: 1551–64.

32 Hannah M, Hannah W, Hodnett E. Planned caesarean section versus planned vaginal birth at term: a randomised multicentre trial. *Lancet* 2000;**356**:1375.

33 Duley L, Neilson JP. Magnesium sulphate and pre-eclampsia. *BMJ* 1999;**319**:3–4.

34 Gülmezoglu AM, Duley L. Anticonvulsants for women with eclampsia and pre-eclampsia: a survey of obstetricians in the United Kingdom and Ireland. *BMJ* 1998;**316**:975–6.

35 Smith A, Hatcher J, Mackenzie I *et al.* Randomised controlled trial of treatment of chronic suppurative otitis media in Kenyan school children. *Lancet* 1996;**348**:1128–33.

36 Mabey D. Importance of clinical trials in developing countries. *Lancet* 1996;**348**:1113.

37 Lumbiganon P, Hofmeyr J, Gülmezoglu M, Pinol A, Villar J. Misoprostol used in the third stage of labour is associated with pyrexia and shivering. *Br J Obstet Gynaecol* 1999;**106**:304–8.

38 Duley L. Maternal mortality and hypertensive disorders of pregnancy in Africa, Asia, Latin America and the Caribbean. *Br J Obstet Gynaecol* 1992;**99**:547–53.

39 Duley L. Magnesium sulphate versus diazepam for eclampsia. In: *Oxford Database of Perinatal Trials.* Version 1.2, disk issue 4. Oxford: Oxford University Press, 1990.

40 Duley L. Magnesium sulphate versus phenytoin for eclampsia. In: *Oxford Database of Perinatal Trials.* Version 1.2, disk issue 4. Oxford: Oxford University Press, 1990.

41 Duley L. Magnesium sulphate regimens for women with eclampsia: messages from the Collaborative Eclampsia Trial. *Br J Obstet Gynaecol* 1996;**103**:103–5.

42 Mahomed K, Garner P, Duley L. Tocolytic magnesium sulphate and paediatric mortality. *Lancet* 1998;**351**:293.

43 Department of Health, Welsh Office, Scottish Office Department of Health, Department of Health and Social Services, Northern Ireland. *Why mothers die. Report on confidential enquiries into maternal deaths in the United Kingdom 1994–1996.* London: TSO, 1998.

6 Improving the quality, number and progress of randomised controlled trials

ROBIN J PRESCOTT, CARL E COUNSELL,
WILLIAM J GILLESPIE, ADRIAN M GRANT,
IAN T RUSSELL AND SUSAN ROSS

Improving the quality, number and progress of randomised controlled trials was the subject of a recent systematic review commissioned by the United Kingdom National Health Service Research and Development Health Technology Assessment Programme.[1] As this chapter draws heavily on results from that review, it is worth summarising its methodology. This differs appreciably from the conventional systematic review of a particular health technology in several important ways. Firstly, there is the enormous volume of literature potentially relevant to the review. The initial search strategy yielded 66 000 hits on MEDLINE for a five year period. Thus the review could be systematic, but it could not aim to be comprehensive. Another difference from conventional systematic reviews is that the type of evidence is different. Often a systematic review would be interested in results from randomised controlled trials, and anything that was not a controlled trial would be rejected. There are surprisingly few randomised studies of randomised trial methodology, and so a wider range of study designs was considered for this review. Information on trial methodology may be incidental to the reporting of trial results. Surveys may be conducted of trials or trialists. There may be reports of secondary research on trial methodology. Useful data may come from systematic reviews of treatment. Even educational articles have to be considered, as many aspects of clinical trial design and analysis are not based on quantitative data, but on the power of logical argument.

The review is thus different in concept to many systematic reviews. In order to synthesise the results, the topic was broken down into different areas: design issues; barriers to participation in randomised trials; limiting factors related to the conduct and structure of trials; analysis; limiting factors relating to the reporting of results; and costs. In each area the objectives were to form recommendations for practice and recommendations for further research. This chapter focuses on some selected recommendations for practice, and does not attempt to deal with areas of analysis or cost.

Trial design issues

Randomisation

A robust randomisation scheme is pivotal in any trial. There should always be a clear protocol for:

- the preparation of the sequence generation
- the method for concealment of a patient's allocation until irrevocable trial entry
- ensuring that the operation of this system does not include any staff involved in determining entry of patients to the trial.

The importance of the concealment of randomisation has been illustrated compellingly by Schulz and colleagues.[2] They found that trials with inadequate concealment of randomisation produced odds ratios for treatment effects that were exaggerated, on average, by 30% to 40%. The results of Moher and colleagues based on 127 trials in 11 meta-analyses replicate this finding.[3] The required security is provided by a telephone or computer-based randomisation scheme, and, as these methods also allow systematic checking of entry criteria, their use is recommended whenever possible.

Patients

The factors that influence which patients become trial participants are:[4]

- patient factors (inclusion and exclusion criteria)
- institutional factors (which centres participate)
- physician preference
- patient consent.

The literature shows a divergence of views on the desirability of permissive or restrictive entry criteria. Arguments in favour of restrictive criteria usually focus on the concept of forming homogeneous groups of patients, and on possible gains in power if between-patient variation is decreased.

The authors are, however, persuaded that, in most cases, permissive entry criteria are preferable for reasons of:

- increased availability of patients, and hence increased power
- reduced trial costs per patient
- greater applicability of the trial results.

Following Collins and colleagues,[5] there is support for the "uncertainty principle" that "the fundamental eligibility criterion is that both patient and doctor should be substantially uncertain about the appropriateness of each of the trial treatments for the particular patient".

The institutional factors referred to above are often reflected in hospital-based trials being conducted in teaching hospitals with little or no district general hospital input. Widening input has been reported as beneficial in cancer trials in the United States.[6] The systematic review[1] recommended that "the clinicians entering patients into multicentre trials should be chosen to give representative patient populations, subject to their having relevant skills and resources to administer the trial treatments and procedures, and having an adequate throughput of appropriate patients".

Sample size

Nobody professionally involved in clinical trials will doubt the fundamental importance of a sufficiently large trial. As discussed in Chapter 5, so called "mega trials" are sometimes essential to establish relatively small but important effects in the treatment of common diseases, as Peto and colleagues have illustrated.[7] The reality is, however, that in some clinical areas large patient populations are not available, while in others it may not be possible to find funding for a mega trial. In some areas, particularly those where there is a continuously distributed primary outcome variable, sample size calculations may show that only a moderately sized trial is needed. There is a problem though when there is a disparity between the desired sample size, and the sample size that can be achieved. It is usually better to conduct a small randomised study than not to do a randomised study at all. However, it must be stressed that such trials should be reported as hypothesis forming rather than hypothesis testing and their data should contribute to an appropriate meta-analysis, made easier by preregistration of trials if the results are unpublished.

Recommendations in this area follow those of Fayers and Machin.[8]

- Sample size calculations should consider a sensitivity analysis, and should give "ballpark" estimates rather than unrealistically precise numbers.
- When only small trials are feasible, they should be reported as hypothesis forming.
- Clinical trials should be preregistered, to allow unpublished results to be traced.
- Full details of sample size calculations should always be reported.
- Funding bodies, independent protocol review committees, and journal editors should all demand provision of sample size considerations.

Run-in period

The desirability, or otherwise, of a run-in period during which the patient receives a non-randomised treatment, prior to formal trial entry and randomisation is an area of controversy amongst trialists. Those with strong pragmatic views will argue against a run-in period on the grounds that the results of trials should reflect what would happen in clinical practice in the non-trial situation. One of the elements in assessing how well a treatment regimen performs is its acceptability, and the level of non-adherence to a therapy is an important component of its evaluation. If a run-in period is used to exclude non-adherers from the trial, then the resulting trial will lack generalisability. On the other hand, if a trialist takes a more explanatory standpoint, the use of the run-in period to exclude non-adherers can increase power. This benefit is particularly marked when an appreciable proportion of participants is expected to be treatment intolerant or fails to comply well enough to achieve appreciable treatment benefit.[9] The well known Physicians Health Study[10] is a convincing example of the possible value of a run-in period, with 33 000 subjects in the run-in phase being reduced to 22 000 for the randomised phase of the trial.

One survey looking at the use of run-in periods reported the surprising finding that very few of the trials employing run-ins assess the level of compliance.[11] The central goal of the run-in is usually to establish a population with stable disease. If adherence is assessed during the run-in, it raises the interesting possibility that this might be used in the analysis of the trial. As a covariate that is likely to be associated with the outcome measures, this suggests that an analysis of covariance may give a useful gain in power.

Barriers to clinician participation

A successful clinical trial will need the cooperation of both patients and clinicians. Table 6.1 indicates some of the principal barriers to clinician participation and gives a concise summary of approaches to overcome these barriers. Time constraints emerged as a reason for physicians not entering a randomised clinical trial of surgery for breast cancer as long ago as 1984, in the United States of America.[12] In the United Kingdom, reforms to the National Health Service within the past decade have exacerbated the problem, and lack of time has been reported as the main disincentive to potential trialists.[13] This is illustrated strikingly by the results of a survey of consultant members of the British Thoracic Society.[14] Respondents were asked to score each of 13 potential factors that might deter them from entering patients into British Thoracic Society projects, which are almost always clinical trials. A six point scale from 0 to 5 was used, with 0 labelled as "no deterrent" and 5 as "definite deterrent" and the intermediate values unlabelled. The results for selected factors are shown in Figure 6.1. Competition with other demands on time emerged as the main deterrent by a substantial margin, with over half of the respondents choosing the "definite deterrent" category. The mean scores for the deterrent factors ranged from 1.2 to 4.0, with the second highest response of 2.7 arising from the factor "forms too complicated/time consuming".

A resolution to the problem of inadequate time cannot be achieved by trial design alone, nevertheless, it is clear that there is a need for designs that make the impositions on the clinician as minimal as possible. Within the United Kingdom, at least, part of the solution must be managerial, with participation in randomised trials being recognised within the United Kingdom National Health Service as a component of the core activity of clinicians.

Table 6.1 Barriers to clinician participation in trials, and recommendations to overcome them.

Barrier	Recommendation
Time constraints	- trials should be a core activity - minimal demands should be imposed
Staffing and training	- preparation and support staff needed
Rewards and recognition	- appropriate (non-financial?) rewards - due credit in publications
Doctor–patient relationship	- minimise research/practice differences
Concern for patients	- minimise burden
Loss of autonomy	- pragmatic trials more acceptable
Protocol	- simple entry criteria - minimal data - relevant/important question with pragmatic design

Trials are commonly run in everyday clinical settings, often without additional support. Apart from the obvious exacerbating effect that this has on time pressures, a lack of research experience[15] and training[16] have been found to be a barrier to patient recruitment. A lack of available support staff, for example clinical trial nurses, has also been blamed for poor recruitment.[16,17]

The impact of rewards for clinicians taking part in trials is difficult to identify. Anecdotally, the authors have found that this has influenced participation in trials in some clinical areas, though the rewards have always been institutional, rather than personal, and have been used to "buy in" the necessary support referred to above. The British Thoracic Society survey[14] did not reveal "nothing in it for me" to be an important deterrent (Figure 6.1), suggesting high levels of altruism. Nevertheless, we feel that clinicians should be rewarded appropriately and adequately for taking part in randomised trials. The rewards need not be financial, but should include positive feedback and support, with contributions credited in all publications and recognised during career progression.

Clinicians' concern for patients has been reported as a barrier, both directly and in terms of the impact on the doctor–patient relationship. The main issues highlighted have been clinicians' difficulties in admitting that they did not know which treatment was best, and the perceived conflict between their roles as clinicians and researchers. Direct concern for patients has focused on treatment toxicity or side effects, and the burden of the trial including travel and

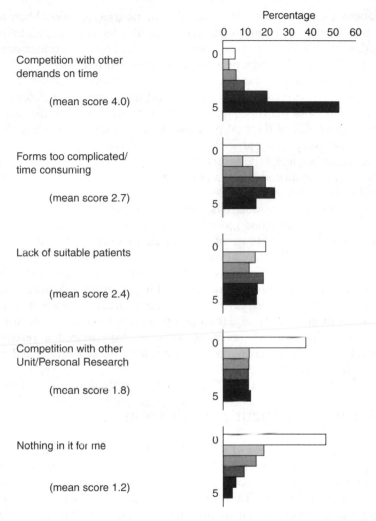

Figure 6.1 Responses by British Thoracic Society consultant members to the deterrent effect of selected factors on participation in multicentre studies.
Note: Possible scores to each factor are 0 (no deterrent) to 5 (definite deterrent).

cost. These barriers can be addressed by designing studies that minimise differences between research and clinical practice, and address questions of sufficient importance for clinicians to be comfortable with the need for the research role. Trials should seek to minimise the burden for patients, both for the benefit to the patient, and to reassure clinicians. Pragmatic trials are most likely to satisfy the above requirements. They are also likely to be helpful in addressing the loss of clinical autonomy implied by trial participation, since this type of design permits more clinician freedom.

Trial design can deter clinician participation in other ways. Overcomplicated forms were the second most important deterrent factor in the British Thoracic Society survey (Figure 6.1). Incompatibility of the trial protocol with normal practice has also been identified as a barrier.[17] Randomised trials are less likely to encounter barriers if the protocol has simple entry criteria, minimal data requirements, and is of a pragmatic design to answer a relevant and important question.

The above discussion has implicitly regarded clinicians as a relatively homogeneous group with the recommendations equally applicable to all. This is, of course, an oversimplification of the situation and is illustrated by another aspect of the British Thoracic Society survey.[14] A comparison of respondents working in district general hospitals with those in teaching hospitals showed that the former group experienced an even greater deterrence to participation because of demands on their time and complicated forms, while those in teaching hospitals experienced a relative lack of suitable patients, and conflicts with other institutional or personal research.

Barriers to patient participation

The ultimate success of a trial depends on patient participation, and there is an appreciable literature detailing potential barriers. The way to overcome some barriers is self apparent, and the first two barriers listed in Table 6.2 come into this category. Patient preferences for particular treatments, or avoidance of placebo may pose a more intractable barrier. There is no easy solution. The possible benefits and adverse effects of the treatment options should be described in a balanced way, together with the rationale for random allocation when the best approach is not known. No coercion should be used, however, to persuade patients to participate and the arrangements for care of those who choose not to participate should be part of the study protocol. The trial design should take into account why patients might refuse participation. For example, change in medication should be minimised, the use of placebo

Table 6.2 *Barriers to patient participation and recommendations to overcome them.*

Barrier	Recommendation
Additional demands of study	- keep demands to minium
Costs to patient	- reimburse
Treatment preference	- present pros and cons
	- discuss rationale for randomisation
	- no coercion
Worry about uncertainty	- public education
Concern about information	- ethical considerations paramount
	and consent

must be justifiable both scientifically and ethically, and the process of randomisation should be presented as an extension of standard medical practice. Nevertheless, a substantial proportion of patients will be concerned by the uncertainties implicit in clinical trial participation. A community survey conducted in the United Kingdom found that 55% of respondents would find it upsetting to be asked to participate in a randomised trial.[18] There is therefore a considerable task of public education to remove the prejudice and anxieties which surround trials.

The way in which information about a study is presented to patients and consent obtained is an important part of trial design and may have profound effects on recruitment,[19] and even on response to treatment or the reporting of side effects.[20] It should go without saying that ethical considerations must remain paramount, but determination of what form of wording is ethical or unethical is subjective. There has been at least one case reported of a centre refusing to participate in a trial because the information provided would frighten patients[17] and, in one survey of European clinicians, 12% reported that they did not inform patients prior to randomisation, despite the protocol.[21]

Conduct of randomised trials

A wide range of issues relating to the conduct of trials may influence their progress and quality. Within this chapter, we will focus on just two topics of major importance: recruitment and compliance.

Recruitment

It is commonly quoted that around half of clinical trials do not achieve their projected sample size. In one survey of a cohort of 41 randomised trials in the United States of America, one third did reach the target, while another one third recruited less than 75% of the planned number.[22] The recommendations that arose from the systematic review[1] are summarised in the box below.

Recommendations for recruitment strategies

- Pilot studies are necessary before starting most trials to check that recruitment strategies are adequate.

- Multiple recruitment strategies should be used with the aim of screening at least twice the planned sample size.

- Recruitment should be closely monitored and there should be contingency plans if fewer patients are randomised than expected.

- Staggering recruitment may help to prevent falling recruitment over time.

- Multicentre trials should not be restricted to expert academic centres.

- Large trials should not be required to register details about those who are not randomised but recruitment logs can be useful and should be encouraged whenever feasible, especially in pilot trials or trials in rare conditions.

Pilot studies are considered by some to be particularly important, not merely to assess the logistics of what occurs after randomisation, as is conventional, but to ensure that estimates of eligible subjects and recruitment strategies are adequate. A contentious issue is the use of recruitment logs, on which some trialists take entrenched but opposed positions. In mega trials the need for simplicity dictates that recruitment logs to register details of those not randomised should not be employed. They can, however, be valuable in smaller trials, especially perhaps in pilot studies to aid with planning the major study, and in rare diseases where they can help in studying the epidemiology of the disease and management policies outside the trial.

Compliance

Compliance, as indicated in the earlier section on run-in periods, is not commonly assessed, even in situations where it is relatively easy to do so. When it is assessed, most of the methods used, based upon the returned medication, tend to overestimate compliance. Sophisticated monitoring of the use of inhalers, for example, has identified patients who discharge their inhalers repeatedly before clinic visits after infrequent previous use. This type of white coat compliance, either by destroying unused medication or taking the medication only when a clinic visit is due will usually be undetectable, as sophisticated monitoring is rarely possible because of cost. Thus, methods such as tablet counts may not be totally reliable, but in a double-blind study, should at least give an unbiased comparison of compliance on alternative medication. If compliance with a particular treatment is poor within a trial, this is of course likely to reflect behaviour outside the trial setting. Consequently, from a pragmatic viewpoint, the level of compliance can be seen as one aspect of the assessment of treatment, rather than as a factor which, in an explanatory trial, distorts the effect of treatment. Findings on compliance from the systematic review are presented in the box below.

Findings on compliance

- Poor compliance reduces the power of a trial.

- Compliance is rarely assessed.

- Interviews, pill counts, diaries overestimate compliance.

- White coat compliance can occur, just before assessments.

- Sophisticated methods may not be practical.

Reporting of randomised trials

One of the fascinating facts to emerge from recent research on the reporting of efficacy and effectiveness data is that the way results are presented influences how clinicians respond to the information. Relative benefits are more likely to be acted upon than the same information presented as an absolute benefit, while, if the absolute benefit is presented as "number needed to treat", it is even less likely to be acted upon.[23] There is a need therefore to present differences between trial treatments in both absolute and relative terms.

The quality of the reporting of trials has been observed to be poor in numerous surveys over a variety of clinical conditions. To our knowledge, no survey has found *any* trial feature to be consistently well reported and some features such as the sample size and method of randomisation have been reported very badly. In the review we did identify four surveys which found that quality was improving over time, but there were also four surveys which did not show this. Of greatest concern is the drawing of conclusions which are not supported by the data. For example, 12% of positive findings were unsupported by the data in one review of 61 trials evaluating non steroidal anti-inflammatory drugs.[24]

Ongoing issues

In conclusion, we will consider some of the ongoing issues facing trialists today, on which it is possible to take an optimistic view of the future.

CONSORT guidelines

The CONSORT (Consolidated Standards of Reporting Trials) guidelines[25] provide a standardised framework for reporting trials. The need for such guidelines is overwhelming, as discussed in the previous section. Anecdotal evidence leads to the conclusion that they have had a very salutary effect on clinicians who might, in the past, have been tempted to hide some of the less robust aspects of their trial in the small print. CONSORT does achieve greater transparency. Although guidelines will always benefit from some refinement, and regular evaluation is essential, generally these have been welcomed as a very positive move that seems certain not only to improve the reporting of trials but also to have a knock on effect on their conduct.

Cluster randomised trials

Issues about cluster trial methodology are becoming increasingly common in the major medical journals. This highlighting of the method has brought with it an increasing realisation that standard methods of analysis are inappropriate. The end result of recognising this is that the analyses presented in very recent articles are usually exemplary.

Ethics committee review

In the United Kingdom we are in a period of evolution. Irreconcilable differences were prone to emerge between ethics committees in their responses to the same multicentre trial. This led to the present system in which trials involving five or more hospitals are initially assessed by a Multicentre Research Ethics Committee. Following approval by this Multicentre Committee, the proposal is considered by Local Research Ethics Committees. These Local Committees can only deal with matters of local implementation, rather than fundamental design issues. This well motivated scheme has generated delays in getting trials started, and can result in voluminous paperwork.[26] The really encouraging feature is that these problems are being recognised at the highest levels and steps are being taken to streamline the system. At the time of writing, the Central Office for Research Ethics Committees (COREC) within the United Kingdom National Health Service is in its infancy. In the British Thoracic Society survey referred to earlier, one respondent commented "the effort of getting two [British Thoracic Society] projects turned down has deterred me from further effort". It is anticipated that such situations will become a thing of the past.

References

1 Prescott RJ, Counsell CE, Gillespie WJ *et al.* Factors that limit the quality, number and progress of randomised controlled trials. *Health Technol Assess* 1999;**3**:No. 20.
2 Schulz KF, Chalmers I, Hayes RJ, Altman DG. Empirical evidence of bias. Dimensions of methodological quality associated with estimates of treatment effects in controlled trials. *JAMA* 1995;**273**:408–12.
3 Moher D, Pham B, James A *et al.* Does quality of reports of randomised trials affect estimates of intervention efficacy reported in meta-analyses? *Lancet* 1998;**352**:609–13.
4 Begg CB. Selection of patients for clinical trials. *Semin Oncol* 1988; **15**:434–40.
5 Collins R, Peto R, Gray R, Parish S. Large-scale randomised evidence: trials and overviews. In: Wetherall DJ, Ledingham JGG, Warrell DA, eds. *Oxford Textbook of Medicine, Vol 1, 3rd ed.* Oxford: Oxford University Press, 1996:21–32.

6 Hunter CP, Frelick RW, Feldman AR *et al*. Selection factors in clinical trials: results from the Community Clinical Oncology Program Physician's Patient Log. *Cancer Treat Rev* 1987;**71**:559–65.

7 Peto R, Collins R, Gray R. Large-scale randomised evidence: large, simple trials and overviews of trials. *J Clin Epidemiol* 1995;**48**:23–40.

8 Fayers PM, Machin D. Sample size: how many patients are necessary? (editorial review). *Br J Cancer* 1995;**72**:1–9.

9 Schechtman KB, Gordon ME. A comprehensive algorithm for determining whether a run-in strategy will be a cost-effective design modification in a randomised clinical trial. *Stat Med* 1993;**12**:111–28.

10 Buring JE, Hennekens CH. Cost and efficiency in clinical trials: the US physicians' health study. *Stat Med* 1990;**9**:29–33.

11 Lang JM. The use of a run-in to enhance compliance. *Stat Med* 1990;**9**:87–95.

12 Taylor KM, Margolese RG, Soskolne CL. Physicians' reasons for not entering eligible patients in a randomised clinical trial of surgery for breast cancer. *N Engl J Med* 1984;**310**:1363–7.

13 Smyth JF, Mossman J, Hall R *et al*. Conducting clinical research in the new NHS: the model of cancer. United Kingdom Coordinating Committee on Cancer Research. *BMJ* 1994;**309**:457–61.

14 Hetzel MR, Lee T, Prescott RJ *et al*. Multi-centre clinical respiratory research: a new approach? *J R Coll Physicians Lond* 1998;**32**:412–16.

15 Winn RJ, Miransky J, Kerner JF, Kennelly L, Michaelson RA, Sturgeon SR. An evaluation of physician determinants in the referral of patients for cancer clinical trials in the community setting. *Prog Clin Biol Res* 1984;**156**:63–73.

16 Shea S, Bigger JT Jr, Campion J *et al*. Enrolment in clinical trials: institutional factors affecting enrolment in the cardiac arrhythmia suppression trial (CAST). *Control Clin Trials* 1992;**13**:466–86.

17 Penn ZJ, Steer PJ. Reasons for declining participation in a prospective randomised trial to determine the optimum mode of delivery of the preterm breech. *Control Clin Trials* 1990;**11**:226–31.

18 Corbett F, Oldham J, Lilford R. Offering patients entry in clinical trials: preliminary study of the views of prospective participants. *J Med Ethics* 1996;**22**:227–31.

19 Bergmann JF, Chassany O, Gandiol J *et al*. A randomised clinical trial of the effect of informed consent on the analgesic activity of placebo and naproxen in cancer pain. *Clin Trials Meta-Analysis* 1994;**29**:41–7.

20 Myers MG, Cairns JA, Singer J. The consent form as a possible cause of side effects. *Clin Pharmacol Ther* 1987;**42**:250–3.

21 Williams CJ, Zwitter M. Informed consent in European multicentre randomised clinical trials – are patients really informed? *Eur J Cancer* 1994;**30A**:907–10.

22 Charlson ME, Horwitz RI. Applying results of randomised trials to clinical practice: impact of losses before randomisation. *BMJ* 1984;**289**:1281–4.

23 Bucher HC, Weinbacher M, Gyr K. Influence of method of reporting study results on decision of physicians to prescribe drugs to lower cholesterol concentration. *BMJ* 1994;**309**:761–4.
24 Rochon PA, Gurwitz JH, Simms RW *et al.* A study of manufacturer-supported trials of nonsteroidal anti-inflammatory drugs in the treatment of arthritis. *Arch Intern Med* 1994;**154**:157–63.
25 Begg C, Cho M, Eastwood S *et al.* Improving the quality of reporting of randomised controlled trials. The CONSORT statement. *JAMA* 1996;**276**:637–9.
26 Al-Shahi R, Warlow CP. Ethical review of a multicentre study in Scotland: a weighty problem. *J R Coll Physicians Lond* 1999;**33**: 549–52.

7 The nuts and bolts of doing a clinical trial

EIVIND BERGE AND PETER SANDERCOCK

Most medical interventions have only moderate effects. To detect such moderate benefits reliably requires trials with large sample sizes,[1] and to achieve this within reasonable time and at reasonable cost requires a large collaborative group of clinicians. The protocol has to be simple, there should be a secure and preferably central randomisation system, and the design should employ the most efficient means of collecting and managing data. A well planned close out at the end of recruitment is important to get follow up data as complete and accurate as possible. Finally, the results should preferably be reported in a high impact journal in the name of the collaborative group as a whole, which rewards the collaborators for all of their efforts (provided the journal lists all the active contributors to the trial). Clinical trial management therefore involves team building and requires a variety of skills to "keep the show on the road".[2]

The nuts and bolts of doing a clinical trial

- A collaborative group.

- Simple and efficient trial design.

- Secure (preferably central) randomisation.

- Efficient data collection and management.

- Well planned close out, with complete and accurate follow up data.

- High impact presentation and publication.

Building the collaborative group

A successful trial is driven by a burning clinical question. If clinicians find the research question important, they are more likely to want to be involved in the trial and to donate of their time and effort. Since large scale non-commercial (or "academic") trials generally involve collaborators putting in their effort for little or no money in return, the trial design has to be simple and efficient, so that the trial procedures do not take up a lot of the clinician's time.

Building the collaborative group

- Trial addresses a burning question.
- Simple and efficient trial design.
- Charismatic lead trialist.
- Collaborators treated with respect and made to feel valued.
- Trial has an "identity".
- Regular collaborators' meetings.
- Support for travel, training, and meetings.

The lead trialist has an important role in establishing and maintaining the collaborative group. It is hard to define the personality traits of the ideal principal investigator, but it certainly helps if he or she has a degree of "charisma" and the ability to motivate the group. Other characteristics may be equally important too. The lead trialist should have the ability to make the collaborators feel valued, and that their contribution, however small, is still important, and that the trial as a whole is at "the cutting edge of medical research". The trialist is dependent on the collaborators, so the trial coordinating team should always treat them with respect, paying attention to their viewpoints and responding quickly to their needs.

The collaborative group works best if it has an "identity", and an easily recognisable and attractive trial name and logo is important in this respect. Collaborators' meetings are an important part of building the trial "identity" and esprit de corps. Of course, they also offer opportunities to inform the collaborators of the trial's progress and to discuss problems arising from the trial. Collaborators welcome the open discussion that can occur in such meetings, which is often lacking in international conferences. Working together in a trial in this way often involves forging interdisciplinary links, getting people to work together who have not done so in the past, and this has the potential to enrich and stimulate the collaboration.

The International Stroke Trial[3] showed that this formula works. The unanswered burning question at the start of the trial was: "should patients with acute ischaemic stroke have aspirin, heparin, both, or neither?" This question, and the trial's simple design, excited a sufficiently large number of clinicians (across 4 continents, 36 countries, and 467 hospitals) to enable the study to recruit its target of 20 000 patients. At the same time, Chinese colleagues were doing the Chinese Acute Stroke Trial[4], so providing – together with the International Stroke Trial – evidence on the effects of aspirin in 40 000[5] and heparin in 20 000[3] randomised patients.

How to get started

Trials of this scale can be completed on a surprisingly small budget; the International Stroke Trial cost less than £1 500 000. The trial started recruitment without a formal grant, as many trials do. It began in 1991 with 33 centres in a "start up phase" which recruited 984 patients over the first two years. During this phase the procedures were simplified and made more efficient. The two years also allowed the group to recruit new centres and countries to be ready for the main phase. The trial was funded with interim support from the Clinical Trial Service Unit in Oxford, and £25 000 from the aspirin manufacturer. Once it became clear that the trial was feasible and recruiting well it was possible to persuade the Medical Research Council to award a grant for the main study. In this way the start up phase could just roll on into the main phase of the trial without losing momentum. A "pilot study" that is finished off and reported separately from the main study risks a loss of momentum, and you then have to start all over to get the main trial up and going.

It is often the case that trials do not attract large scale grants until they have proved that it is possible to randomise a sufficient number of patients. In other words, trials must get started with randomisation somehow or other, and "pull themselves up by their bootstraps", attracting more funding as they become more successful. The CRASH (Corticosteroid Randomisation After Significant Head Injury) trial of corticosteroids for head injury[6,7] began in a similar way. The "start up" feasibility phase was funded by a small grant from the Medical Research Council and a donation from a pharmaceutical company. This "start up" phase recruited well and achieved good follow up, which facilitated the process of obtaining grant funding for the main phase. The CRASH trial has now launched into a 20 000 patient study.

Central randomisation systems

One of the keys to a high quality trial is a secure central randomisation system.[8] Doctors will always want to try to make sure that their patients get new and exciting treatments, and, even within a randomised trial, doctors may want to influence the treatment their patients receive.[9] They want to see the allocation list, they will try to persuade the telephone operators to reveal the next treatment allocation, and so on. Doctors are well meaning and they want the best for their patients, but this often subverts the trial randomisation.[9]

It is possible to do trials without central randomisation and to use methods that minimise the risk of randomisation being subverted, but for brevity we will limit our discussion to centralised randomisation systems. In its most simple form, you need a random allocation list and a reliable person (who is not responsible for recruiting patients) to receive the randomisation telephone calls. This could be someone who is working on some other aspect of the trial, but who is always

---

Simple centralised randomisation system

- A random allocation list (on paper or computer).
- A reliable person from coordinating centre, not responsible for recruiting patients.
- A means of communicating with the clinician wishing to enter a patient.
- A mechanism to ensure that the next treatment allocation is kept secure until needed.

---

available to handle telephone calls requesting randomisation. When the investigator telephones the trial office or faxes the randomisation form to enter a patient, the operator needs to first record the baseline details and then, when they are complete, give out the next treatment allocation. To make sure that the treatment allocation is kept secure until it is needed, the operator must be well trained to reveal the treatment allocation only to clinicians wishing to enter a patient into the trial and only after baseline data are recorded. Operators must never reveal the allocation for the subsequent patient.

A simple system operating in normal working hours (nine am to five pm, five days a week), will be sufficient for interventions that are not very time dependent, for example randomisation to local or general anaesthetic for patients having elective, non-urgent carotid endarterectomy. A better nine to five system uses a computer to generate the next allocation, instead of paper randomisation lists. This allows collection of baseline data and stratified or adaptive randomisation (minimisation).[10]

For more urgent interventions, like thrombolysis for acute ischaemic stroke or new treatments for heart attack, you may need randomisation systems available 24 hours a day, seven days a week. Even this system can be made to work without access to expensive randomisation services. You need a staff member with a "randomisation kit" who can receive telephone calls out of hours. For a simple trial this can be a mobile telephone and a palmtop computer. For a more complex trial it might be an automated system with more complicated hardware, intelligent telephone software such as CallSuite, and a database that is running at all times. In the FOOD (Feed Or Ordinary Diet) trial[11] stroke patients are allocated to different means of feeding on a 24 hour basis, using an automated randomisation system (Figure 7.1). Clinicians wanting to randomise patients telephone the trial office, and are automatically connected to a computer. The computer is programmed with voice prompts given by the principal investigator, asking for the patient's name and other patient details. These are then keyed in on the telephone pad, and the computer generates a treatment allocation and sets off a voice message, telling the next treatment allocation to the clinician. In case of technical problems (for example, when the main randomisation computer "freezes" or crashes: not an uncommon experience) a back up system is also important, which could pe provided by a member of the trial team with a mobile telephone and a palmtop or laptop randomisation system. Automated randomisation systems can also be done over the internet. The VITATOPS (VITAmins TO Prevent

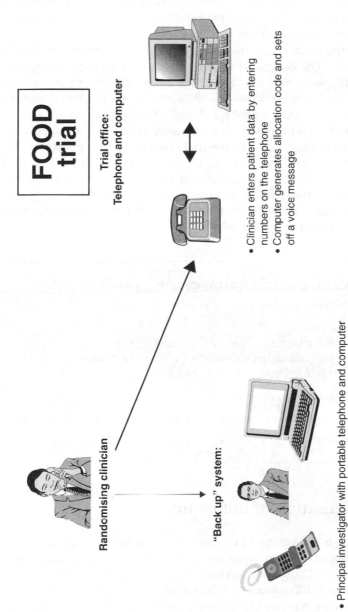

FOOD trial

Trial office:
Telephone and computer

- Clinician enters patient data by entering numbers on the telephone
- Computer generates allocation code and sets off a voice message

Randomising clinician

"Back up" system:

- Principal investigator with portable telephone and computer

Figure 7.1 Automated central randomisation system in the FOOD trial.

Stroke) trial of vitamins for stroke prevention[12] has its own randomisation page on the world wide web. Once you have entered a password and the patient's baseline data, the next treatment allocation is generated and sent back to you.

A secure central randomisation system does not need to be hugely expensive. The basic nine to five system with a randomisation list costs effectively nothing. The more advanced nine to five system based on a computer costs less than £1 000 for hardware, and the hardware and software for the "gold" 24 hour system are around £3 500. A "home made" central randomisation system also has other advantages. It allows the trial team to build rapport with the collaborators as the system can be modified to meet their needs if there are problems. You can record your own sound files, so that the clinician hears the familiar voice of the principal investigator, and you can achieve 24 hour access, which can be very important for recruitment into the trial.

Advantages of "home made" randomisation systems

- Low cost
  - basic system: almost no extra cost
  - more advanced system: < £1 000 for hardware
  - "gold" system: < £3 500 for hard-/software.

- Trial team builds up rapport with collaborators.

- You can record your own sound files for the automated system.

- Access 24 hours a day, seven days a week (good for recruitment).

Maximisation of follow up

A trial is no use if you do not get follow up data. Patients with head injuries, such as those included in the CRASH trial, are often young men. Those who survive often have cognitive impairment or behavioural difficulties, so when they get a postal questionnaire they may be reluctant to complete and return it. Many therefore doubted that the trial would ever achieve more than a 60% follow up rate. Edwards and Diguiseppi, and others from the CRASH office at the Institute of Child Health in London, are undertaking a Cochrane systematic review of randomised trials of interventions to improve the completeness and quality of follow up.[13] They found 300 trials, some of which have tested interventions on a very large scale. For example, the use of an incentive to return the questionnaire has been tested in 76 trials with a total of 84 000 subjects. Some trials tested whether monetary incentives work, and found that they do. Other trials tested whether you should put money in the envelope or send it as a reward *after* the person has returned the questionnaire, and found evidence in favour of putting the money in the envelope. The evidence also supports the use of stamps, rather than putting the letter through an automatic franking machine. Each trial needs to develop efficient systems to obtain complete follow up data from the patients randomised.

Conclusions

Clinical trials are a most powerful tool in clinical research. Much of the collective practical wisdom about how to make trials succeed has until now been passed on by apprenticeship, but is now being gathered together in a more formal way. This book and other information sources should, we hope, lead to more trials being done, and done efficiently, so that they answer the "burning questions" reliably.

References

1 Yusuf S, Collins R, Peto R. Why do we need some large, simple randomised trials? *Stat Med* 1984;3:409–22.
2 Warlow C. How to do it. Organise a multicentre trial. *BMJ* 1990;**300**: 180–3.
3 International Stroke Trial Collaborative Group. The International Stroke Trial (IST): a randomised trial of aspirin, subcutaneous heparin, both, or neither among 19435 patients with acute ischaemic stroke. *Lancet* 1997;**349**:1569–81.
4 CAST (Chinese Acute Stroke Trial) Collaborative Group. CAST: randomised placebo-controlled trial of early aspirin use in 20,000 patients with acute ischaemic stroke. *Lancet* 1997;**349**:1641–9.
5 Chen ZM, Sandercock P, Pan HC *et al*. Indications for early aspirin use in acute ischemic stroke: a combined analysis of 40 000 randomised patients from the Chinese Acute Stroke Trial and the International

Stroke Trial. On behalf of the CAST and IST collaborative groups. *Stroke* 2000;**31**:1240–9.

6 Yates D, Roberts I, on behalf of the CRASH trial management group Corticosteroids in head injury. It's time for a large simple randomised trial. *BMJ* 2000;**321**:128–9.

7 Corticosteroid Randomisation After Significant Head Injury. www.crash.lshtm.ac.uk (accessed 11 Jul 2001).

8 Torgerson DJ, Roberts C. Understanding controlled trials. Randomisation methods: concealment. *BMJ* 1999;**319**:375–6.

9 Schulz KF. Subverting randomisation in controlled trials. *JAMA* 1995;**274**:1456–8.

10 Roberts C, Torgerson D. Randomisation methods in controlled trials. *BMJ* 1998;**317**:1301.

11 The International Stroke Trials Collaboration. The FOOD trial (Feed Or Ordinary Diet trial). www.dcn.ed.ac.uk/food/(accessed 11 Jul 2001).

12 Vitatops, VITAmins TO Prevent Stroke. www.health.wa.gov.au/vitatops/(accessed 11 Jul 2001).

13 Edwards P, Clarke M, Diguiseppi C, Roberts I, Pratap S, Wentz R. Methods to influence response to postal questionnaires [protocol]. In: Cochrane Collaboration. *Cochrane Library*. Issue 4. Oxford: Update Software, 2000.

8 Building resources for randomised trials

BARBARA FARRELL AND PATSY SPARK

The human and financial resources for doing randomised trials are finite, so it is crucial that every effort is made to ensure that good ideas can be developed simply and efficiently into high quality studies. In their chapter Elvind Berge and Peter Sandercock point out that much of the collective wisdom about doing trials has been passed on by apprenticeship, and Robin Prescott and colleagues highlight some of the barriers to conducting trials. This chapter will summarise some of the processes and resources necessary for the efficient conduct of trials, and will suggest ways to facilitate sharing of knowledge and expertise about how to do trials.

Little has been written about how to set about the process of developing a question or hypothesis into an actively recruiting randomised trial. There are no clearly defined operational models to follow, but there is a wealth of anecdotal experience that should not be lost. Experienced trialists will have put together, either formally or informally, checklists of essential steps in the development of a trial,[1] based on their experience of what works and what does not work. However, those planning their first trial have to start from scratch, unless they are lucky enough to have access to a trial office, or someone with relevant experience. Many trials struggle to get underway because the people running them have not been able to find information about the best processes for establishing and delivering a trial. Figure 8.1 illustrates that these processes can be complex. A trial needs to be managed from its inception, like any other business. There are a relatively small number of trial offices around the world which successfully roll out one high quality trial after another. But, there are many, many other groups and individuals who have a burning desire to do it themselves. They want to add to our knowledge of how to provide better health care, and should be able to rapidly find the support that they need.

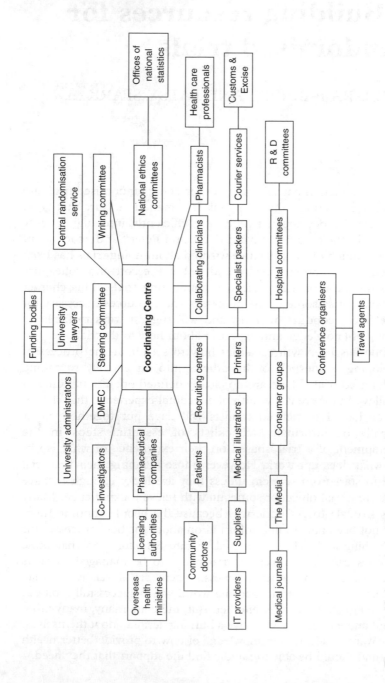

Figure 8.1 Various relationships in the development of randomised trials.
Note: DMEC: Data Monitoring and Ethics Committee; IT: information technology; R&D: research and development.

How to plan a trial

There are a few things to think about before you start.

- How will the protocol be developed?
- Who needs to be involved in the early stages of development?
- If additional funds are needed, where will they be sought?
- How will data be managed?

Justify the need for the trial

A good trial takes a lot of hard work. To demonstrate that this effort is worthwhile, and motivate others to contribute, you first need to justify the need for the trial.

- What is the scale of the problem? How common is the condition and how serious?
- Has the question already been answered? What are the results of a recent systematic review?
- How are clinicians currently managing the problem? Is there a recent survey of practice?
- Is the intervention feasible? Is there sufficient clinical uncertainty, and variation in practice?

Develop the protocol

The detailed methods for conducting a trial are set out in the protocol checklist (see Box). Deciding how the trial will be conducted and the data will be analysed is crucial in reducing bias. The protocol is the scientific justification for the study and the project plan. It also plays a crucial role in securing ethics approval and funding. Protocol development can take a long time to do well, often years for large studies. Consultation with everyone likely to be involved in the study is crucial, for example, doctors, nurses, general practitioners, consumers, statisticians, and health economists. The best advice for someone planning their first trial is to look at some successful protocols. Try to get hold of two or three protocols on different topics to get a feel of what approaches would suit your study. Many are now available on the world wide web, or just telephone the coordinating centre and ask for a copy.

Protocol checklist

- Title.
- Summary.
- Background and rationale for the trial.
- Hypothesis to be tested.
- Primary outcome(s).
- Secondary outcomes.
- Inclusion and exclusion criteria.
- Interventions to be tested.
- Estimated sample size.
- Information for patients and consent.
- Analyses plan, including dummy tables.
- How patients will be entered into the study, concealment of allocation.
- Duration and methods for follow up.
- Data collection, including questionnaires.
- Trial management.
- Trial supervision.
- Publication policy.
- References.

The protocol should be easy to read, precise, and unambiguous. It should set out clearly the data to be collected, the outcomes to be measured, and how the analysis will be conducted. Any analysis not specified in the protocol is hypothesis generating rather than hypothesis testing. Clear descriptions of how the trial will be managed, supervised, and analysed ensure that the conduct of the trial is transparent.

Sample size

The sample size is calculated based on the primary outcome. It is an estimate of how many people would need to be in the trial to demonstrate, with prespecified power and statistical significance, the smallest effect that would be clinically important. Often it is sensible to calculate a range of estimates, based on a variety of possible frequencies for the primary outcome in the control arm, and a range of possible effects. For large trials, this estimate will be reviewed by the data monitoring committee, which has confidential access to the trial results.

Inclusion and exclusion criteria

These should be clear and explicit. For large pragmatic trials it is also important that they are simple,[2] and inclusive, rather than exclusive.

Randomisation and concealment of the allocation

Randomisation means that chance is the only factor that determines which allocation each participant receives. The most important factor for secure randomisation is concealment of the treatment allocation; the allocation must be concealed until after the person has been entered into the trial. It should not be possible to guess or find out the next treatment allocation. Common methods for concealment of the allocation include central randomisation by telephone, fax, email or on the internet, and use of consecutively numbered and sealed boxes or envelopes.

How patients will be entered into the study

The procedure for entering patients into the trial must be easy, so as not to burden busy clinicians. It also needs to be realistic and practical, for example telephone randomisation is no use if participating centres do not have reliable access to telephones! Other factors to consider are where and when will participants be recruited, and who will explain the trial and randomise participants. The information to be collected before trial entry should be kept to an absolute minimum.

Data collection forms

The data collection forms should start being designed early in the process of protocol development. They should be designed so that they collect all the information in the format required by the dummy tables, which will provide the basis for the trial analysis. Information not included in the dummy tables should not be part of the data collection. This takes considerable discipline, but will avoid omissions in the data collection and minimise the collection of data that is never reported.

Simple tips for the design of data forms

- Always collect raw data, if necessary it can be categorised later.
- Build in cross checks for important times and dates.
- Ask questions in an order that will make sense to the person completing the form.
- Line up boxes, to reduce the risk of any being missed.
- Make the forms look attractive, don't clutter them up or use too small a font.
- Get professional advice, for example from your local medical illustration department.

Apply for ethics approval

Ethics committee approval is required before recruitment can start. These committees have a range of both clinical and lay members, and are guided by the Declaration of Helsinki.[3] The application for ethics approval will need to include final copies of the patient information leaflet, consent form, data collection forms, any letters to general practitioners or trial participants, and any promotional material to be seen by the public.

Apply for funding

Most trials will need some external funding; the amount will vary depending on factors such as the size of the study and how much is available within the institution. There are a wide range of sources for funding, and many agencies have websites with instructions for applicants and forms. Also, on the world wide web there are various databases of funding bodies, which can be searched by topic and type of research supported.

Develop a collaborative group

To be successful, most trials depend on developing a collaborative group. For large trials this will be a diverse multidisciplinary group

Funding application checklist

- Coordinating office: trial manager, programmer, data manager, secretary
  - consider whether full or part time, and when to start and finish.

- Other input: statistician, health economist, consumers, research fellow
  - consider how much input and when needed.

- Randomisation system.

- Intervention: drug, placebo, packaging, distribution.

- Computing: hardware, software, computer consumables.

- Printing costs: protocols, data forms, posters, newsletters.

- Postage: freepost for return of questionnaires, multiple mailshots.

- Telephone/fax/email: sufficient to maintain regular contact with all centres.

- Consumables: stationery, telephone, postage, photocopying, freepost licence.

- Centre costs (if applicable): telephone, photocopying, secretarial/nursing support.

- Travel: site visits, collaborators' meetings.

- Meeting/travel costs: management group, steering committee and data monitoring committee.

including representatives from each participating hospital. For smaller and single centre studies the group will be less formal, and may be just a small group of like-minded people.

The *Oxford English Dictionary* defines collaboration as "an understanding or contract between individuals". The aim of a collaborative group is to be inclusive rather than exclusive, so being proactive in raising awareness about the project and in inviting people to join the group is important. This can be done, for example, through personal contact, conferences, mailshots, newsletters from the professional colleges, and journal articles. If a survey of practice is being carried out among clinicians, it is simple and cheap to include a question in the survey asking whether or not they are interested in collaborating on a trial.

A trial is likely to be more successful, and enjoyable, if members of the collaborative group feel they "own" the project. This ownership will be fostered by involvement and consultation at every stage, from protocol development to publication of the results. In the past, consumers have often been excluded in the planning of trials, or have had their role restricted to commenting on patient information leaflets and the final results. Many research groups have now discovered for themselves that welcoming consumers into their collaborative group greatly enhances the project. Many consumer groups have a particular interest in promoting understanding of trials, for example Consumers in NHS Research,[4] who facilitate lay collaboration in clinical trials within the United Kingdom National Health Service.

Develop efficient trial management procedures

Once the protocol is developed, it needs to be put into practice: a huge task about which little has been written.[5] This phase will be much easier if trial management has been planned within the protocol, and properly budgeted for. A randomised trial is a business. A trial is often a major investment of both time and money, and should therefore be treated as such and planned with precision. Every trial needs to develop a management plan, and ideally this process should begin within the protocol. It can then be modified and refined, as necessary, as the trial progresses.

The management plan should include an outline of the arrangements for supervision and monitoring of the study, including the steering committee, data monitoring committee, and how day to day running of the trial will be planned and managed. It should also describe who will be responsible for essential activities, such as staff recruitment, communication with the collaborative group, monitoring of recruitment, trial coordination, data management, and awareness raising. The management plan should set achievable targets, provide the framework for building an enthusiastic and efficient team, and detail and justify the necessary resources for delivering a successful trial.

Trial managers have, in recent years, become a highly valued profession, and they have now begun to develop better ways of disseminating and sharing the experience and expertise gained over years of learning on the job. Societies and associations of trial managers in Europe and North America[6,7] are beginning to network and make their knowledge available via the internet, and through journal publication.[4]

Develop efficient systems for trial coordination and data management

A trial, particularly a large trial, needs systems and procedures to monitor every aspect of the study. A systematic approach is needed to monitor recruitment, randomisation procedures, stock control, data management and cleaning, and filing of the collected data. Every piece of paper that relates to a person in the trial should be logged and tracked through the trial office. There needs to be logical and transparent structure, concise documentation, and accountability. If the trial is international, these systems should take into account differing clinical practices and working environments.

Good quality data depends on, amongst other things, effective trial management. Collecting information on a form and entering it on to a computer is simple. However, ensuring that these data are sensible, reliable, and reflect the "truth" is a complicated and detailed process. With the aid of computers, data validation and quality control can be quick and efficient. Whenever possible, trials should be managed with the most up to date electronic systems (Figure 8.2). These systems also need to be flexible and adaptable, so that they can be tailored according to the needs of the people collaborating in the trial. In a multicentre trial, particularly one involving centres in a wide range of settings, such flexibility may be critical for success.

Most modern trials will use computerised systems for trial management and data management. Such computerised systems are wonderfully efficient for keeping track of recruitment, data collection, and for recording who has been sent what within a study. For large trials this may be a customised programme, but smaller studies may adapt off the shelf software. Asking the advice of an experienced trial programmer can be invaluable in helping to make the right decisions for a new trial.

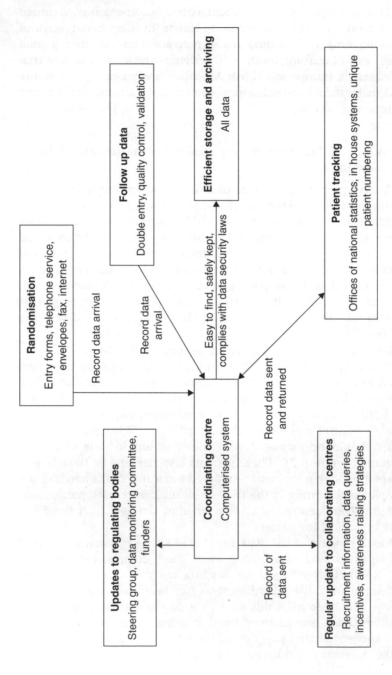

Figure 8.2 Flow chart for computerised systems for randomised trials.

The design of any customised database needs careful consideration, and should undergo wide consultation and piloting. The database, and programming, may have to last several years and a good design will save endless trouble and effort later in the trial. Randomised trials rarely run as originally planned and the needs of the trial also change over time, so the flexibility to modify the database is important. The choice of which software to use may not be easy. Factors to consider are whether it can cope with the expected number of records, how easy it would be to make changes, how confidentiality will be ensured, and whether it can handle data for the analysis.

Clinicians are usually fitting the trial into their already busy workload. It is essential, therefore, that the trial procedures can be integrated into their existing practices, minimising any additional workload. It is the role of the trial coordinating centre, and efficient trial management procedures, to take the burden off the clinicians. Trials must not overload those clinicians willing to participate. Consequently, there is a great deal of work for the coordinating team. Efficiency is paramount and good robust systems are essential.

Market the trial

A trial needs to be marketed from inception, and the box outlines some of the processes involved. This list is a guide only, as marketing needs to be tailored to the needs of the individual study. If in doubt, it is often worth trying something to see if it works, and if it doesn't work – change it. If nobody knows about the trial it will not attract collaborators, sponsors or participants. A clinical trial is a very odd commodity to manage or "sell." Clinical trials need to be packaged in ways that will offer some sort of kudos or recognition to those willing to participate. As described in Chapter 7 this means, in effect, establishing and promoting a "club" to develop an "esprit de corps".[8] This can involve delicate, sometimes controversial, management and marketing skills and, as described earlier, these negotiations should start at the protocol development stage, or earlier. Marketing need not be expensive, but including things like newsletters and collaborators' meetings in your budget will let funders know you mean business.

Marketing a trial checklist

At the protocol and funding stage

- Choose a good acronym.

- Budget for marketing costs, such as newsletters, collaborators' meetings, headed notepaper.

- Develop partnerships with consumer groups, invite their comments on the protocol and budget for their ongoing input.

- Start developing the collaborative group.

At the start up and recruitment stage

- Choose a striking logo, and put it on a letterhead and all trial materials.

- Write articles for medical journals and consumer conferences.

- Present papers and posters at relevant conferences.

- Provide user friendly, attractive, and stylish trial materials along with clear guidance on how to use them.

- Be proactive and inclusive in encouraging people to join the collaborative group.

- Visit centres, meet and talk to as many of those involved in the trial as possible.

- Consider a 24 hour on call service for dealing with trial queries.

- Consider a launch meeting for collaborators.

- Consider a dedicated trial website.

To maintain recruitment

- Circulate regular newsletters with updates on progress.

- Use posters or letters of congratulation to acknowledge good progress.

- Consider offering incentives for achieving targets, such as T shirts, mugs or pens.

- Consider focused collaborators' meetings, bringing together people who work in the same region or country.

- Use opportunities to "piggy-back" small meetings on to national or international conferences.

- Visit centres where there are particular difficulties.

Ensure compliance with appropriate regulations and regulatory bodies

Clinical trials need to comply with current data protection laws and Good Clinical Practice (GCP) guidelines.[9] This information is not always easy to come by, and there have recently been substantial changes in the regulatory framework for trials. The full implications of these changes for trials within the United Kingdom are still being clarified. When the implementation guidelines are available they need to be widely disseminated and kept up to date, for example by funders, in journals, and on the internet.

Develop a publication policy

Planning dissemination and how credit for the trial will be shared are also important components in planning a trial. For collaborative trials it is vital that appropriate credit is given where it is due. This will often mean publication of the results as a collaborative group, or by a named few on behalf of the collaborative group. Contributorship for the collaborative group should then be listed at the end of the paper. In a large trial, inevitably there will be people who made substantial contributions but who, for reasons of space, cannot be named. Certificates of collaboration for those who made a substantial contribution to the trial, but who are not named on the paper, can be an effective way of making everyone feel that their contribution is valued.[10]

The trial means little if results are not disseminated and taken into account in clinical practice. Commonly used ways of making the results of a trial widely available include articles in medical journals, trial registers, systematic reviews (such as *The Cochrane Library*[11]), and conference presentations. Dissemination should also include consumers, for example, through reports and articles in the lay media and consumer journals. Advantages of multicentre trials are that each collaborator can be responsible for local dissemination.

Trial results should be published, whether or not they show a difference, and it has been described as scientific misconduct not to publish.[12] Reporting of results should maintain confidentiality, and it must not be possible to identify either individuals or centres within the report. Individual participants can only be identified with their written permission. As discussed in Chapter 6, CONSORT[13] provides a structure (Figure 8.3) for improving the transparency of trial reports.

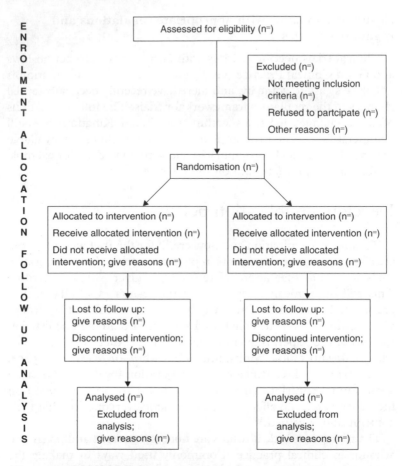

E
N
R
O
L
M
E
N
T

A
L
L
O
C
A
T
I
O
N

F
O
L
L
O
W

U
P

A
N
A
L
Y
S
I
S

Assessed for eligibility (n=)

Excluded (n=)

Not meeting inclusion criteria (n=)

Refused to partcipate (n=)

Other reasons (n=)

Randomisation (n=)

Allocated to intervention (n=)
Receive allocated intervention (n=)
Did not receive allocated intervention; give reasons (n=)

Allocated to intervention (n=)
Receive allocated intervention (n=)
Did not receive allocated intervention; give reasons (n=)

Lost to follow up: give reasons (n=)
Discontinued intervention; give reasons (n=)

Lost to follow up: give reasons (n=)
Discontinued intervention; give reasons (n=)

Analysed (n=)
Excluded from analysis; give reasons (n=)

Analysed (n=)
Excluded from analysis; give reasons (n=)

Figure 8.3 CONSORT flowchart.

Facilitating sharing of knowledge and expertise in trials

Recurring themes in this book are the need for those planning and doing trials to have reliable and rapid access to the expertise they need, and for development of ways that avoid reinventing of the wheel. Barriers to such access are often geographical location, time, lack of funding, or just uncertainty about where to look or who to ask.

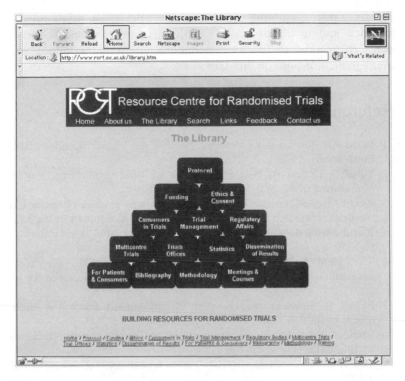

Figure 8.4 The Resource Centre Library website.

The Resource Centre for Randomised Trials[14] is one recent initiative that is trying to tackle some of these issues. The Centre has a range of activities, including developing a programme of workshops designed to help people tackle issues encountered within their own studies. A key component of the Resource Centre is a web-based library (Figure 8.4). This aims to provide a user friendly interface for accessing information relevant to trials. For example, the library has links to other websites, such as those of funding agencies and databases, consumer groups interested in trials, ethics committees, and regulatory agencies. It also provides checklists for trials, with examples of trial materials such as protocols, consent forms, and patient information leaflets. A constantly changing database of meetings, courses, and specific workshops relevant to trials is also available. The aim of the library is to classify, and thereby make more accessible, the vast and rapidly growing amount of information relevant to trials on the internet, and to fill any gaps identified in this process. Overall, the Centre aims to facilitate collaboration in the conduct and management of high quality trials.

References

1 Jadad AR. *Randomised Controlled Trials: a user's guide*. London: BMJ Publications, 1998.
2 Yusuf S, Collins R, Peto R. Why do we need some large, simple, randomised trials? *Stat Med* 1984;**3**:409–20.
3 World Medical Association. Recommendations guiding physicians in biomedical research involving human subjects. As adopted by the 18th World Medical Assembly, Helsinki, June 1964 (the "Declaration of Helsinki").
4 The Help for Health Trust. Consumers in NHS Research. www.hfht.org/ConsumersinNHSResearch/index.htm (accessed 11 Jul 2001).
5 Farrell B. Efficient management of randomised controlled trials: nature or nurture. *BMJ* 1998;**317**:1236–39.
6 Clinical Trial Managers Association. www.ctma.org.uk (accessed 11 Jul 2001).
7 The Society for Clinical Trials. www.sctweb.org (accessed 11 Jul 2001).
8 Warlow CP. How to do it: organise a multicentre trial. *BMJ* 1990;**300**: 180–3.
9 International Conference on Harmonisation for Good Clinical Practice (ICH GCP) 1996. www.ncehr-cnerh.org/english/gcp
10 Duley L. Anonymity of authorship. *Lancet* 1995;**345**:1372.
11 Cochrane Collaboration. *Cochrane Library*. Oxford: Update Software, 2001.
12 Chalmers I. Under-reporting research is scientific misconduct. *JAMA* 1990;**263**:1405–8.
13 Moher D, Schulz K, Attman D for the CONSORT Group. The CONSORT statement revised recommendations for improving the quality of reports of parallel-group randomised trials. *Lancet* 2001;**357**:191–4.
14 Resource Centre for Randomised Trials. www.rcrt.ox.ac.uk (accessed 11 Jul 2001).

9 The role of data monitoring committees

RICHARD DOLL

The history of randomised controlled trials was examined a couple of years ago on the 50th anniversary of the publication of the Medical Research Council's streptomycin trial, the first example of the modern type of randomised trial.[1] Since then, further attention has been paid to the history of the subject. Iain Chalmers (personal communication) has found that several people had, in one way or another, used or proposed randomisation previously. There can be no question, however, about the origin of the modern randomised trials in the two studies that Bradford Hill and his colleagues organised shortly after the Second World War. The first was actually a prophylactic trial of immunisation against whooping cough, but the results were not published until after those of the streptomycin trial for pulmonary tuberculosis, which has consequently been regarded as the first. In retrospect, it is now quite clear that the methodology was introduced to eliminate selection bias, not for any esoteric statistical reason.

Early methods for monitoring trials

Over the next 10 years randomised trials gradually began to be used by physicians generally, first of all in the United Kingdom and then in the United States and Scandinavia; but it was a long time before they were commonly used in most of the other European countries. At first, the trials were mostly small, being carried out by single physicians. For example, I conducted several to test different therapies for peptic ulcer.[2] But when more patients were needed than one physician could get from his own practice, committees were set up that encouraged 10 or 20 physicians to come together and collaborate in the conduct of a trial. I say physicians, because the extension to surgery and obstetrics came somewhat later. These committees ran trials much like the modern ones, except that the numbers were smaller. If they had a few hundred patients in the trial they thought they were doing well.

There were no data monitoring or ethics committees for a trial in those days. If the clinician running the trial was wise he consulted a statistician before he began, rather than presenting him with the results to analyse later. But with the trials that were run by committees (for example those run by the Medical Research Council, for the treatment of, say, leukaemia, rheumatoid arthritis, or ulcerative colitis) where you needed a number of clinicians to get together to have enough patients, then there was some more formal organisation. There was a statistician to the committee, a clinician who was organising it acting as scientific secretary, who preferably was not admitting patients himself, and a senior clinician in the chair. The statistician and the secretary of the committee kept an eye on the results and told the chairman if they thought that there was any reason for stopping the trial. In fact, there very seldom was, because nearly all the trials showed, at the best, only moderate effects and ran for as long as they had been funded. It seldom happened that there was any clear reason for stopping, either because of adverse effects or for clear benefit seen with the relatively small numbers that were likely to have been admitted. So there wasn't usually much of a problem about whether to stop a trial or to continue it.

The only time I remember a problem was in a trial in which the first four deaths all occurred in patients on a new treatment, cortisone, for severe ulcerative colitis. Had the next death occurred in that group we should have stopped the trial. Actually the next death did not and the trial ended by showing that cortisone was in fact beneficial.[3] Since then I have had a similar experience on a number of occasions, i.e. a treatment appearing to have an adverse effect initially and then turning out to have a benefit. So monitoring committees have to keep cool, knowing that some extraordinary findings may turn up when the total number of patients entered is still small. Looking at the results as they came in, as we used to do, created the further problem that a P value of 1 in 20 would turn up fairly frequently. This was, of course, appreciated and Peter Armitage tried to deal with it by introducing a technique of sequential analysis, which allowed one to look at the results after each patient was treated.[4] It required patients to be paired and the decision taken whether one member of the pair did better, worse, or the same as the other. The technique was not, however, widely used and it was realised that it was better not to keep checking the results, but to analyse them periodically at stated intervals; the fact that they were analysed several times could be taken into account when interpreting the P values.

The first data monitoring committee

Trials proceeded like this, reasonably satisfactorily for many years, but with few exciting discoveries. Trouble started, however, when funds for medical research began increasing, because many people began to carry out trials and conflicting results came to be reported, as they invariably will be when the numbers in each trial are small. This could be dealt with in two ways. One was a competent combination of the results of all trials, by what is now called a meta-analysis. This technique was introduced into the United Kingdom by Richard Peto for the trials of aspirin in the treatment of myocardial infarction[5] and independently, in a less developed form by Tom Chalmers in the United States, for the trials of anticoagulants for the same condition.[6] Meta-analysis was, however, a novel idea when it was first introduced and clinicians did not fully appreciate what it was doing. Consequently they didn't take much notice of its findings. It was, therefore, fortunate that shortly afterwards Richard Peto and his colleague Rory Collins found an opportunity for dealing with the problem in a second way, by organising a really large trial that would give a definitive result.

The first such large trial was carried out to test the effect of atenolol, a β-blocker given intravenously. This trial, which became known as ISIS-1, recruited 16 000 patients from 245 coronary care units in 16 countries.[7] With this trial the need for a specific, independent, data monitoring committee became clear. One was consequently set up and, as it happened, I was asked to chair it. No particular problem arose. We looked at the results every six months or so and there was never any reason for stopping the trial. Ethically there was no real problem about introducing it either, but the ethics were the responsibility of the initial ethical committee. In this case there was only indirect evidence that the treatment might be of benefit and there was some concern that it might, in certain circumstances, be hazardous. The decision whether to use it was really unclear (a so called grey area) for everyone. The results showed that there was a small reduction in vascular mortality during the seven day treatment period from 4.6% (controls) to 3.9% (atenolol) which was just statistically significant (P<0.04).

When to stop a trial

The next trial was very different, both in its justification and in its results.[8] ISIS-2 made the data monitoring committee face up to the real ethical problem of deciding when it was to report to the steering committee. I say report to the steering committee because, in my opinion, data monitoring committees should not stop trials or authorise their continuation. That is the responsibility of the people that are running the trials. What a data monitoring committee has responsibility for is telling the steering committee what the results are when they think the steering committee should know them. It is then up to the steering committee to decide what to do.

One problem that was highlighted was an ethical issue relating to membership of the data monitoring committee, which concerned specifically the views of the members of the committee when the study began. Now, as it happened, I was chairing that committee and I told the organisers that if I had a myocardial infarction I wanted to have both the special treatments under test: namely, streptokinase and aspirin. I was not willing to be a subject of the trial, because I was confident that both of the treatments were beneficial. How then could I chair the data monitoring committee? Without any difficulty, in my view and that of the trial organisers, because all the information that had led me to conclude that both these treatments were effective was made available to the doctors admitting the patients, and through them to the patients entered into the trial. The question was the confidence you had in meta-analyses. As far as aspirin was concerned, the result of the meta-analysis was, to me, quite clear; but to the great majority of doctors it obviously was not. You couldn't, they thought, have a beneficial effect on the risk of myocardial infarction by doing something so simple as giving an aspirin, which had been given for headaches for the previous 50 years, so doctors were just not prescribing it. I went to a meeting of cardiologists at which the use of aspirin was discussed and asked those to hold up their hands if they were prescribing aspirin, and about 5% did.

This was why we wanted to do the trial, even though Richard Peto and Rory Collins, who originated the trial, and I, who chaired the data monitoring committee, were all quite convinced that aspirin was beneficial. The only way that we were going to get patients to be given aspirin was by demonstrating its value in a large randomised trial, and the same applied to the use of streptokinase. The difficulty with the latter was not that doctors didn't think that it was ever beneficial, but because it occasionally caused cerebral haemorrhage. If the clinicians had seen such a case, or had a friend who had had such a case, they reacted by thinking the treatment was too dangerous and ignored the findings of the meta-analysis, which, on balance, showed that the benefit was much greater than the risk. So there we were on a monitoring committee, most if not all of us wishing to have one or both of the special treatments if we were to have a myocardial infarction.

So what should we have done about reporting to the steering committee? It was no good just reporting straight away that aspirin and streptokinase had beneficial effects, because the reason for doing the trial was that most cardiologists were not taking any notice of the information that was already available. What we were to do was determined by our terms of reference: namely, to report to the steering committee when, in our opinion, the trial evidence, combined with any other new evidence that had been reported since the trial began, would be sufficient to bring about a change of practice if reported to the profession in general. There is no particular P value for that. It certainly wasn't 0.05; it might have been somewhere near 0.001, but we didn't actually set ourselves a specific value.

The decision when to report was a qualitative one. Was the evidence that we progressively gained from the trial going to be sufficient to change practice? After a time we decided that the evidence of benefit from streptokinase, if given within six hours of the onset of the disease, was so strong that, if reported and published, it would change practice. We consequently reported the results to the steering committee; but they didn't stop the trial. The members of that committee thought that the trial should go on, that the evidence was not strong enough to convince all cardiologists, and the fascinating thing is that when the trial findings were reported to all the participating clinicians, recruitment *increased*. Unbelievable, perhaps, but that was the way it worked out; presumably because many of the clinicians, particularly in Scandinavia, had not been giving streptokinase because they thought it was too hazardous. All our report had done was to make them think that there might be something in the treatment after all. So, despite having reported to the steering committee results which, in our opinion, were sufficient to change medical practice, it hadn't done so, except insofar as it got more clinicians to enter patients into the trial.

A few months later the results became even clearer and there was evidence of benefit from streptokinase up to 12 hours after the onset of the disease. We reported the further findings and the trial was stopped. Practice now did change and within a few months surveys showed that some 90% of clinicians were using streptokinase, instead of the original 5%.

So far I have not mentioned the results with aspirin. As it turned out, aspirin did not actually show clear evidence of benefit in the early stages of the trial. Eventually the evidence was very strong indeed and the data monitoring committee was publicly criticised for not having reported on aspirin earlier. We could not be criticised for not reporting on streptokinase, as we had reported on that quite early; but we were criticised for not reporting on aspirin. In fact, much of the trial evidence of benefit from aspirin turned up in the patients whose outcome was notified after the trial had been closed. We had not had clear results for aspirin in front of us. The P value for benefit from aspirin was of the order of 0.05 when we reported the findings on streptokinase, and the trial was closed. As the final results came in, however, aspirin was suddenly shown to be clearly beneficial and to have reduced fatality to much the same extent as streptokinase had. Moreover the benefits of the two treatments proved to be additive.

In my view the ethical responsibility of the data monitoring committee, for the sort of large trial that I have been describing, is not to the next patient to be admitted to the trial; that is the responsibility of the clinician who decides whether to admit the patient or not. The ethical responsibility of the data monitoring committee is to the next thousand patients: to all the patients who are going to suffer from the condition in the years to come. If our responsibility is to those patients, it is to see that they are likely to get the most effective treatment. There is no point in doing a large trial, unless the results, if they show that one treatment is better than another, do, in fact, change medical practice. As far as I am concerned, if I am to be on a data monitoring committee, it is on one condition; we report the results to the steering committee running the study when, in our view, the results, coupled with any other findings that may have been published since the trial began, will be such as to alter practice and bring about a benefit for succeeding generations of patients.

Data monitoring and ethics committees

This fairly simple criterion is complicated now by the fact that sometimes data monitoring committees are set up to be data monitoring *and ethics* committees, and that does create some difficulty. I would prefer to see the original ethical committee continue its responsibility for the ethics of the trial, rather than thrusting this on to the data monitoring committee. But the reality is that the responsibility is now frequently thrust on to the data monitoring committee, and we have to consider what extra responsibility this imposes. It does not, I think, alter the criterion that I have just described, but it does require the committee to make sure that all admitting doctors do tell patients about the evidence that is currently available, so that they can obtain properly informed consent. These large trials may last for several years, from the time they are first started until the time they end. Quite a lot of additional information may come in during this time and it is the responsibility of a data monitoring and ethics committee to make sure that, in the light of continually developing knowledge, patients' informed consent is really informed by the existing knowledge. The combination of these two roles complicates the work of the committee. But, as long as it does not cause the principle to be altered, i.e. that the primary responsibility of the committee is to see that practice is changed (if the results indicate that it should be), then it is possible to marry the two responsibilities. But it is not always easy.

For small trials trying out new treatments, the position is, of course, different. The data monitoring committee, if there is one, or the statistician to the trial, if there is not, will want to report the results to the responsible clinician as soon as they conclude that the findings provide good evidence of either benefit or harm.

References

1 Doll R. Controlled trials: the 1948 watershed. *BMJ* 1998;**317**:1217–20.
2 Doll R. Medical treatment of gastric ulcer. *Scott Med J* 1964;**9**: 183–96.
3 Truelove SC, Witts LJ. Cortisone in ulcerative colitis: final report on a therapeutic trial. *BMJ* 1955;**2**:1041–8.
4 Armitage P. *Sequential medical trials*. Oxford: Blackwell Scientific Publications, 1960.

5 Anon. Aspirin after myocardial infarction (editorial). *Lancet* 1980;
  1:1172–3.
6 Chalmers TC, Matta RJ, Smith H, Kunzler AM. Evidence favouring
  the use of anticoagulants in the hospital phase of acute myocardial
  infarction. *N Engl J Med* 1977;**297**:1091.
7 ISIS-1 Collaborative Group. Randomised trial of intravenous atenolol
  among 16,027 cases of suspected acute myocardial infarction: ISIS-1.
  Lancet 1986;**2**:57–66.
8 ISIS-2 Collaborative Group. Randomised trial of intravenous streptokinase, oral aspirin, both, or neither among 17,187 cases of suspected
  acute myocardial infarction: ISIS-2. *Lancet* 1988;**2**:349–60.

10 Bayesian perspectives on the ethics of trials

RICHARD J LILFORD AND
DAVID A BRAUNHOLTZ

Moral consensus is captured in the language used in society at a point in time.[1,2] In this chapter we show how bayesian and decision analytic axioms can be used to clarify the conditions under which clinical trials can be ethical. The resulting concepts can be captured in language. Thus, under fisherian and Neyman Pearson notions of statistical significance and hypothesis testing, the ethical basis of clinical trials is typically articulated in terms of the "uncertainty principle". However, under bayesian and decision analytical paradigms, reflecting degrees of belief and scales of utility, "uncertainty" is exposed as a very vague and permissive term. "Equipoise" or "indifference" describe a much more precise ethical basis for randomised trials.

The old paradigm

The statistical paradigm guiding the analysis of clinical trials is typically based on hypothesis testing. Thus, the popperian notion of falsification was (arguably inappropriately) carried over into the design and interpretation of clinical trials,[3] investigators set out to test a "null hypothesis". Sample sizes were selected to give pre-specified risks of wrongly, or rightly, rejecting the null hypothesis.[4] The language used to describe and defend trials reflected this concept that trials had dichotomous outcomes, that the null hypothesis would either be rejected or not. Trials were supposed to provide "an answer" to important clinical questions.[5] An under-powered study, which had little chance of rejecting the null hypothesis, even if it was substantially false, was considered "bad science", and hence "bad ethics".[6-9] Interventions were regarded as beneficial, or harmful, only when a null hypothesis had been rejected at a specified confidence level, usually 95%. If the null hypothesis had not been rejected at the required level of precision, then the effects of the intervention should still be regarded as "uncertain"; indeed, a subsequent trial might be needed in order to provide such an "answer" and be justified on this basis.[10-13] So long as one was "uncertain", a clinical trial would be regarded as ethical since future patients would benefit at no net cost to current patients.[14] However, as soon as the threshold of significance was exceeded, and the null hypothesis rejected, randomisation could no longer be said to be as good as any other option from the patient's perspective. "Uncertainty" was dispelled instantly, once statistical significance was reached, and from then on a randomised trial would not be considered ethical.

The gradualist view of knowledge

Our main argument is a simple one; knowledge accrues by degree and, although decisions are dichotomous, knowledge is not. Since knowledge comes in degrees, the term "uncertainty" is equivocal, sometimes meaning one thing and at others, something different.[15] Thus, a clinician can offer a patient entry in a clinical trial on the basis of "uncertainty" simply meaning that the null hypothesis has not been "disproven", while a patient may understand something quite different; namely that each treatment alternative is as likely as the other to be better, or even that the outcome with the greatest chance of occurring is the null result. Similarly, a previous trial result that favours one treatment, but falls short of statistical significance, should nevertheless rationally influence the decision whether or not to participate in a trial. To describe the effects of treatment, both before and after such a result, as "uncertain" is, to say the least, an "economy with the truth". Although this has been pointed out from time to time down the years,[15,16] the effects of treatment are often still described as "uncertain" in the context of trials and, as long as hypothesis testing was accepted as the predominant statistical paradigm, ethical arguments tended to follow the resulting dichotomy of knowledge.

The paradigm of certainty versus uncertainty is no longer so pervasive. Firstly, statisticians have increasingly urged that trials should be used to estimate treatment effects, and not just to test hypotheses in a popperian sense.[17] Thus the use of confidence intervals is widely advocated, with "confidence" usually set at 95%.[18] However, confidence intervals do not indicate how likely it is that a treatment will have a given effect when applied to a patient indistinguishable from those in the clinical trial; confidence intervals still belong to a form of statistics known as frequentist, which deal with the probability of obtaining a dataset, given a certain underlying state of the world, for example that the comparator treatments produce equivalent effects. What clinicians need is the probability of a certain underlying state of the world, such as an effect of a certain magnitude, given the data. Since confidence intervals do not give this type of probability, it is not clear how they should be translated into action. For this reason, a confidence interval is usually described in terms of whether or not it includes a null effect. In other words, as it is not clear how it *should* be interpreted, it is usually "reduced", in effect, to the same hypothesis test of the null hypothesis, which it was hoped and intended to augment and largely replace.

The statistical method that can tell us the probability of certain sizes of clinical effect, given data that have been observed in a trial, is known as bayesian. Bayesian probabilities represent degrees of belief about the state of the world, and so are subjective. Bayesian probabilities can thus describe, for instance, "the probability that the true relative efficacy of drug A compared to placebo is more than k", whereas frequentist probabilities cannot. It either is or it isn't. A consequence of the bayesian view of probability is that the influence of observed data on beliefs comes via "updating" a "prior" distribution of beliefs. Thus, an essential part of bayesian thinking is that of a starting-distribution of beliefs.

If the null hypothesis were the most likely hypothesis in prospect, then the highest point on the distribution would correspond to the null hypothesis (Figure 10.1). If results in either direction are thought increasingly less likely, then a corresponding distribution of prior probabilities could be drawn. This distribution would then be updated by the results of a trial to produce a posterior distribution, as shown in Figure 10.2. The larger the trial, the narrower the posterior distribution becomes.

Note that a frequentist analysis starts with assumptions about the state of the world, assumptions that may be more or less credible. In order to conduct a bayesian analysis, a prior distribution of probabilities reflecting beliefs about the true state of the world is required and again this may be more or less credible. The essential

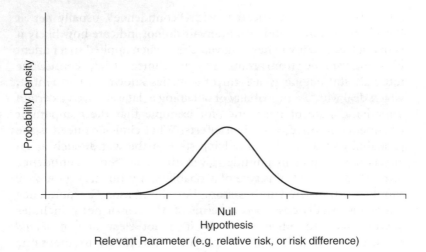

Figure 10.1 Distribution of beliefs when the null hypothesis is the most likely hypothesis. Area under the curve represents probability. Total area under the curve is 1.

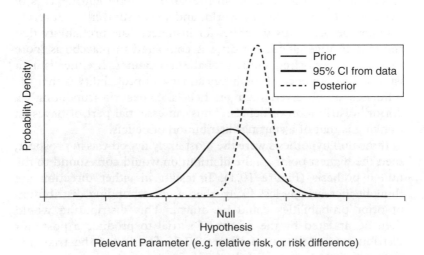

Figure 10.2 Distribution of beliefs updated with the results of a trial, posterior distribution. CI: confidence interval.

point in terms of ethics, however, is that a prior statement of beliefs requires careful consideration of where the truth may actually lie, even in cases where no previous trial evidence exists; a dichotomous view of knowledge is no longer tenable. For example, a number of clinical trials of hormone replacement therapy are currently taking place, to study effects on cardiovascular disease and breast cancer, among other outcomes. A late menopause is associated with breast cancer, while an early menopause, whether iatrogenic or natural, is associated with a lower risk. Breast cancer occurs in a target organ for oestrogen. Preliminary non-randomised studies have suggested there may indeed be a small increase in the risk of breast cancer proportional to the duration of use of hormone replacement therapy. Such information brings into being a picture of the world that is not altogether neutral. While there is still "uncertainty", most people would have a "prior" centred around a, perhaps small, increase in the risk of breast cancer if hormone replacement therapy is taken. Because the bayesian technique requires a "prior", and because bayesian methodology is receiving increasing attention, the notion of prior beliefs, even in advance of a clinical trial, is becoming more accepted. Given the growing acceptance of the mathematical construct of a "prior" amongst influential academics, uncertainty based on anything falling short of $P < 0.05$ seems increasingly inadequate as a moral basis for a trial. In other words, it is now much more starkly obvious that there are degrees of uncertainty, it is harder to ignore this when such degrees of uncertainty are an input into statistical analysis. Put yet another way, as our epistemic stance moves from "yes/no" hypothesis testing to updating the probability density, so our understanding of the ethics of clinical trials, and the language that we use to discuss this, must change.

This chapter thus has its theoretical foundations in bayesian statistics and decision analysis (expected utility theory). Those unfamiliar with these topics will find our analysis difficult to follow and may like to refer to review articles on bayesian statistics[19–21] and decision analysis[22–24].

Should Jill be randomised?

In the remainder of this chapter, we will consider a cancer patient, Jill, and a clinical trial comparing two treatments, A and B. In the first instance, we will consider the scenario in which A and B have equal "costs", both in monetary terms and in terms of known and postulated side effects. We will also assume that Jill is intellectually of sound mind, not in acute distress, and not in need of urgent treatment. First a decision must be made as to whether it is ethical to offer Jill entry into the trial. Even if the trial is ethical, however, this does not mean that Jill should accept randomisation. Although Jill, guided by her doctor and/or on the basis of her own reading, may believe either A or B, to be better; the situation may also arise where her beliefs as to the effectiveness of A and B are evenly balanced. Her "prior" for the difference in mortality might be centred symmetrically on zero. Under these circumstances, Jill will be unable to say which of A or B she prefers, and she might well be prepared to enter the trial. Remember we have assumed, for the moment, that the side effects of A and B are equal. For Jill, the treatments are equivalent in prospect, or using the word coined for the purpose, she is equipoised. Note that simply to say that Jill is uncertain whether A is better than B is a much *weaker* statement. We can now say that a clinical trial is ethical when Jill is equipoised. So, the ethics turn firstly on whether it is reasonable to offer randomisation to Jill and secondly, on how Jill is counselled, since unless Jill is very knowledgeable, whether or not she ends up in equipoise will be heavily influenced by what she is told.

There are, of course, some immediate, theoretical and practical problems here. On the theoretical side, there is the question of whether equipoise can actually exist, given that it is always possible to make a decision if one has to. To put this in more mathematical terms, the centre of mass of any probability distribution is vanishingly unlikely to be at any given point, including the point of equipoise. Since a "prior" is a psychological construct, we think that equipoise has to be operationalised as a psychological phenomenon. It could be thought of in practical terms as the situation that applies when a well informed person, who is acting in his/her own best interests, would be equally happy to receive treatment A or B. Because equipoise also has a mathematical definition some people, while understanding the point we are making, dislike the term equipoise. For them, the term "indifference" may be preferable, since it is explicitly located in the mind of the decision maker, rather than in the realms of mathematics.

However we describe equal expected utilities, the requirement that they should be equal leaves us with a practical problem in that people will rationally be uncertain much more often than they are indifferent. In short, recruitment to trials is likely to be lower if they are ethically constrained by equipoise or indifference, rather than the more permissive notion of "uncertainty".

An attempt to get round the difficulty of reduced entry in trials when they are based on equipoise not uncertainty

Freedman[25] distinguishes between individual equipoise, which he calls theoretical equipoise, and collective equipoise, which he calls clinical equipoise, and which refers to experts collectively, however defined. He goes on to argue that the ethics of clinical trials should be based on collective, not individual, equipoise. His argument, simply stated, is that the duty which clinicians have to their patients is different to that which they may have towards cherished members of their own families. Thus, while individual equipoise is a proper basis for family decisions, clinicians are judged by professional standards. When the profession is equipoised, collective standards are not violated by a randomised trial.

We will leave aside the thorny issue that collective equipoise will seldom be based on a perfect, 50:50, split.[26] Here we argue that collective equipoise impinges on the ethics of trials in two quite distinct settings and that the moral significance of collective equipoise is quite different in each. In short the presence or absence of collective equipoise could be used to:

- guide collective decisions, for example those of ethics committees, as to whether it is ethical for a trial to proceed in the first place; Whether Jill can be offered entry in a trial
- determine what patients are told when they are invited to participate in trials, or whether or not a patient who cannot give consent should be randomised.

In our opinion, the requirement that collective equipoise should exist is appropriate for the decision to allow a trial to proceed. It is also proper to disclose its existence when offering entry in a trial. However, it should not be used to define the limits of what individual patients are told. It is not enough simply to say to Jill "experts are divided on whether A or B is better". We argue that clinicians should not censor further information that might assist patients in deciding whether or not they are in equipoise. Such information might describe the clinician's personal belief and/or it might consist of the information and analysis by which a clinician could derive a personal belief. The point is that the clinician should disclose as much information as possible or practicable to assist autonomous decision making. We argue that such disclosure is necessary to protect trust in all cases and to optimise choice in cases involving trade-offs. If personal equipoise is necessary, then the invitee must be given, or at least offered, all the information that they might need to make up their minds about whether or not they really are "indifferent".

Trust and the need for individual equipoise

Suppose there is collective equipoise, so that faced with Jill's case many clinicians would prefer A, but many others would prefer B. Therefore the ethics committee cannot disallow the trial on the basis that there is already sufficient consensus on the best treatment. Jill's doctor is amongst those that prefer A, but should he or she tell Jill this? Freedman acknowledges that doctors may prefer A and would choose A for themselves or a family member. But he argues that collective equipoise is sufficient for trial entry and that a doctor does not have to treat patients in the same way as a family member, because the doctor is bound only by collective norms.

We, and others,[27] strongly disagree, feeling that it is inherent in the hippocratic concept of trust between a patient and doctor that doctors must do their best for the patient. We further argue that this implies that doctors should disclose their personal beliefs about, and preferences for, the alternative treatments, or offer to do so, and/or provide such data as might exist, and such analysis as may be necessary, for the patient to make up his or her own mind. If Jill has faith in her doctor's abilities, then the doctor's opinion is important evidence for her decision making process, as would be the believed existence of collective equipoise.[16] Jill may want to know what other relevant information exists and engage in discussion about the verisimilitude of such data. The issue of clinician–patient communication, and exactly how much information it is possible or appropriate to give, must vary from circumstance to circumstance and from patient to patient. However, maintaining patients' trust and faith in doctors seems to require that clinicians, when inviting people to be randomised, should disclose or offer to disclose any lack of personal equipoise and/or disclose the basis for different opinions. Potential participants must be able to form their own "prior" and/or have an opportunity to hear their caregiver's "prior".

If a patient is incompetent, for example if he or she is unconscious, and no relatives are in attendance, or if he or she does not wish to take the decision, then it would seem to us that the doctor should treat the patient like a member of his or her own family, and only randomise in the belief that all trial treatments are equally good for the patient, in prospect. We totally reject Freedman's argument that the doctor can rely on collective norms, and hence collective equipoise, in this context.

So far, we have described the situation where no trade-off is required because treatments have similar "costs". A closer look at how a patient might decide whether two dissimilar treatments were equally beneficial, in prospect, helps to clarify the need to go beyond collective equipoise and "uncertainty" when offering patients entry into clinical trials.

Choice, trade-offs, and decision analysis

Decision analysis has provided a formal basis to the concept of patient choice, including the choice to participate in clinical trials. Decision analysis, sometimes called expected utility theory, deals with the much more usual circumstance where trade-offs have to be made between one therapy and another.

Jill might have cancer of the larynx. In that case, it may be fairly certain that radical surgery is more effective than radiotherapy in leading to cure, but a trial may be proposed to measure the extent to which this is so. The "prior" would be centred on an improvement in survival, but it would be quite vague, admitting of many different treatment effects. However, we know up front that surgery has the serious side effect of greatly diminishing (indeed, temporarily abolishing) the power of speech. Thus, there is a trade-off between this side effect and the "prior" estimate of the absolute differences in the life prolonging effectiveness of the two treatments. In such circumstances, the null hypothesis is not only known not to be true, but also, in any case, it doesn't equate to equipoise; it is irrelevant. Decision analysis keeps probabilities and values (measuring the trade-offs that people would make between relevant outcomes) as distinct entities, but combines them to calculate the "worth", or expected utility, of alternative options.[28,29] In this case, it is important to know what a patient would trade off, in terms of longevity, in order to avoid the loss of the power of speech for one year. If, on the basis of a doctor's or a patient's best probability estimate, surgery stood to increase life expectancy by one year, say from four to five years, and if each post-laryngectomy year was "worth" 0.8 of a post-radiotherapy year, then the expected utility of the two therapies would be equivalent, and the patient would be in equipoise, all other things being equal. The expected utility of surgery (EUs) is 5×0.8, which is equal to the expected utility of radiotherapy (EUr) 4×1.0. Of course, all other things would not be equal, since other trade-offs would need to be factored into a full decision analysis. For instance, preference for mode of death may be relevant, and more remote years may have to be discounted to reflect a preference for the years immediately ahead. Nevertheless, the essential point is that the *intention* of treatment should be to maximise a patient's welfare, to maximise expected utility, and the patient is in equipoise or indifferent when the expected utilities of treatments are judged equal.

Decision analysis, in its full, explicit, and rather stark form, is not necessarily the correct counselling method in all circumstances. The point about decision analysis is that it shows the logical structures that lie behind decisions made. Above all, it reconciles preferences and evidence, by giving values and probabilities due weight within a logical framework. Probabilities are, usually, the province of the professional whilst values reflect patient preferences. Since routine clinical practice, i.e. practice not involving clinical trials, should represent our best attempts to portray probabilities and to incorporate values in a way which is sensitive to the circumstances and psychology of the patient, it would surely be totally inappropriate to adopt a different stance when trials are involved. For example, in the absence of a trial, a clinician would be expected to tell a menopausal woman about the possible effects that hormone replacement therapy might have on her risk of breast cancer. In so doing the clinician's "prior" might be disclosed and/or the patient might form her own "prior". Of course, the clinician would do the same for other outcomes, including, for example, any perception of likely benefit or risk of cardiovascular disease. The patient would then need to consider how she felt about these various conditions, and how she may be prepared to trade one off against another.

Exactly the same exchange should take place in the context of a clinical trial, except that a three way choice should follow this: hormone replacement therapy; no hormone replacement therapy; or trial entry. If a patient were undecided whether she wanted to take hormone therapy or not, in other words when, given the limitations of clinical practice, the expected utilities of both treatments appeared the same, then she would be eligible for the trial. Interestingly, it has been shown empirically that providing more information results in less acceptance of randomisation into a hypothetical trial of hormone replacement therapy.[30] As knowledge and acceptance of bayesian statistics and decision analysis spreads, so it will become increasingly unacceptable to say, for instance, that a trial of surgery versus radiotherapy for laryngeal cancer, or of hormone replacement therapy versus placebo for menopause, is ethical as long as there is "uncertainty". Uncertainty is necessary but not sufficient.

What if Jill is altruistic?

Jill might want to help people who find themselves in her predicament in the future, by contributing to knowledge. If she was already equipoised and not of any altruistic impulse, then she contributes at no cost. If she has a strong preference for one treatment or another, then she is unlikely to accept randomisation. However, if she has a small preference she might give up some expected utility, say one month of a Quality Adjusted Life Year, for altruistic reasons. In one sense, of course, she gains utility through the exercise of altruism. She can be randomised provided this benefit is offset against other net losses in prospect; she may simply have factored altruism into her construction of personal equipoise. In the above example, the trial would be the preferred option as long as the expected survival after surgery was between 4 years 10.75 months, and 5 years 1.25 months, everything else being unchanged. Within this range, the expected utility of the trial is actually greater than the alternatives: expected utility of surgery; or expected utility of radiotherapy. We suspect that many patients will not behave altruistically, though some will be almost excessively so. We argue that doctors should not overtly encourage such altruism, especially from vulnerable patients.

What if Jill is unable to give consent? Then it would be wrong to impute atypical amounts of altruism to her, the golden rule applies and Jill's doctor should only randomise her if he or she would do likewise for his or her own mother. This assumes that there is no reason to suspect Jill's values to be different from the doctor's mother's. Randomising Jill when she could not give consent but where an alternative treatment promised greater expected utility than another would be to sacrifice some of Jill's utility to the common good. This is not, we think, how doctors should behave in the context of a trial. It certainly violates what philosophers call the injunction of Kant but, put more simply, it is not how most patients would want to be treated. The literature on this issue has been reviewed elsewhere.[31]

We concede that there are situations where a doctor can override a patient's preferences (uncontrolled epileptics who continue to drive, for example), but contend that clinical trials are not in this category. In the context of trials, we and most patients[31] think the patient's utility comes first and that, if the patient is conscious or competent, he or she must be offered as much information as possible to help make a choice, in other words to decide whether or not he or she is indifferent. If the patient is not conscious or competent, then the doctor must only randomise him or her if, in conscience, he or she thinks that the expected utilities of the comparative treatments are equal.

What about trials as a treatment, will Jill benefit from participating in a trial?

Here we deal with the idea that clinical trials have a beneficial effect over and above any direct effect of treatment. A recent review of the topic concludes, very cautiously, that there may be a benefit from the trial per se and that this is contingent on the extra attention to detail that patients, in all groups, get in trials. This is the well known protocol effect.[32] A trial then potentially offers two benefits quite apart from treatment received; the expected utility of altruism (EUa), as above, and the further putative benefits of participation, probably realised by following the trial protocol, which we call EUp. Let us imagine, in Jill's case, that in the absence of a trial, radiotherapy would be preferred to surgery (EUr > EUs). In that case, assuming 1:1 randomisation, she would prefer a trial provided that: $EUr < 0.5EUs + 0.5EUr + EUa + EUp$.

The trial is acceptable to Jill provided that she is indifferent, or better, between the trial and the favoured alternative. But caution is needed. Firstly, EUa and EUp are probably not large. We have conjectured that many people will have EUa = 0, no altruism at all, and the evidence for a protocol effect (EUp > 0) is not strong,[32] especially under these conditions where treatment is from the same clinician, whether inside or outside the trial. Secondly, there are serious ethical problems with EUp. The Declaration of Helsinki states that patients' care should not be affected by whether or not they decline to participate; and they certainly should not be induced to participate by the offer of better care. This imperative is widely ignored, with justification, where a new and promising treatment is only available within a trial. However, to tell a prospective participant that they may get a benefit from participating in a trial just because treatment is given more carefully within a trial would clearly be unacceptable, because this state of affairs would in itself be unacceptable. In short, we think that EUa and EUp are marginal considerations and that it is safer to present clinical trials to patients in terms of the prior probabilities of the outcomes of the treatments themselves.

Practical implications

It could be argued that, although the epistemological basis of clinical trials is changing, the implications for the recruiting physician and patient are minimal. While we acknowledge that clinical practice is far more "messy" than theoretical conjecture, what actually happens in doctor–patient communication is influenced heavily by the theoretical models that are carried into the consulting room, and these models are changing. We have argued that the very language in which we express ourselves is changing in a way that is altogether consistent with the paradigms of bayesian statistical inference and decision analysis. We think it will become increasingly unacceptable to tell a patient that there is "uncertainty", or to imply that the "null hypothesis" is being tested, when the clinician's "prior" is one that rationally might provoke a treatment preference.

There are a number of direct policy changes that will arise if indeed bayesian statistical inference, and decision analysis, become widely accepted. Firstly, the rate at which people are likely to be recruited to clinical trials will be much less than was possible previously, funders will have to accept this. Indeed, rather than pressurising researchers to recruit all possible patients, it would be more appropriate to question their methods of consent when recruitment was high, especially if dissimilar treatments were being compared, such as surgery versus non-surgical treatments.

Secondly, it should be much more widely understood that the scientific obligation to provide the community with the best evidence is not the same as the obligation of individual clinicians to do their best for their patients. They overlap only when equipoise or indifference applies, but in other circumstances they may well conflict. Hence, it is entirely unrealistic for organisations whose main responsibility is to the public to expect high recruitment rates to trials where effective, but expensive, new technology is assessed after becoming generally available. It would be far better for such technology to be made initially available only within the context of a clinical trial. This way promising new treatments, such as lithotripters and extracorporeal membrane oxygenation, can be responsibly appraised, without expecting clinicians to be the "gatekeepers".

Thirdly, it should be more widely understood that ethically there is no need for a string of medical prognostic factors to act as eligibility criteria for clinical trials; all that is needed is equipoise or indifference. "Priors" for stratification variables should be elicited in advance, and used in any subsequent analysis. There are many successful examples of trials without rigid entry criteria, but with stratified analysis, for example the Medical Research Council European Carotid Surgery Trial.[33]

Finally, as we have described elsewhere,[34] given bayesian methods we should no longer feel constrained by power calculations, since some meaningful, unbiased information is better than none.[35] This is particularly important for obtaining data on rare diseases,[18,21] but is also relevant to individual clinicians who might be unable to recruit the requisite number of patients, but anticipate replication at a later date.[36] Consequently, "underpowered" trials should not be rejected out of hand, as is currently the policy of many ethics committees, since they do not necessarily constitute "bad science" and should not be regarded as unethical on the basis of power alone.[34]

References

1 Habermas J. *The theory of communicative action.* Translated by Thomas McCarthy. Cambridge: Polity, 1987.

2 Habermas J. *Moral consciousness and communicative action.* Translated by Christian Lenhardt and Shierry Weber Nicholsen. Cambridge: Polity, 1992.

3 Senn SJ. Falsificationism and clinical trials. *Stat Med* 1991;**10**:1679–92.

4 Ambroz A, Chalmers TC, Smith H. Deficiencies in randomised controlled trials. *Clin Res* 1978;**26**:280a.

5 Byar DP. The necessity and justification of randomised clinical trials. In: Tagnon HJ, Staquet MJ, eds. *Controversies in cancer: Design of trials and treatment.* New York: Mason Publishing UK, 1979:75–82.

6 Altman DG. Statistics and ethics in medical research – III. How large a sample? *BMJ* 1980;**281**:1336–8.

7 Altman DG. Size of clinical trials. *BMJ* 1983;**286**:1842–3.

8 Freund PA. *Experimentation with human subjects.* London: Allen and Unwin, 1972.

9 Newell DJ. Type 2 errors and ethics. *BMJ* 1978;**2**:1789.

10 Ashby D, Machin D. Stopping rules, interim analyses and data monitoring committees. *Br J Cancer* 1993;**68**:1047–50.

11 Fleming TR. Historical controls, data banks, and randomised trials in clinical research: a review. *Cancer Treat Rep* 1982;**66**:1101–5.

12 George SL, Li C, Berry DA, Green MR. Stopping a clinical trial early: frequentist and Bayesian approaches applied to a CALGB trial in non-small-cell lung cancer. *Stat Med* 1994;**13**:1313–27.

13 Tannock IF, Boyer M. When is a cancer treatment worthwhile? *N Engl J Med* 1990;**323**:989–90.

14 Weatherall DJ. *Oxford textbook of medicine.* Oxford: Oxford University Press, 1987.

15 Gifford F. Community-equipoise and the ethics of randomised clinical trials. *Bioethics* 1995;**9**:127–48.

16 Lilford RJ, Jackson J. Equipoise and the ethics of randomisation. *J R Soc Med* 1995;**88**:552–9.

17 Freeman PR. The role of p-values in analysing trial results. *Stat Med* 1993;**12**:1443–52.

18 Goodman SN, Berlin JA. The use of predicted confidence intervals when planning experiments and the misuse of power when interpreting results [published erratum appears in *Ann Intern Med* 1995;**122**:478]. *Ann Intern Med* 1994;**121**:200–6.

19 Freedman LS, Spiegelhalter DJ. Application of Bayesian statistics to decision making during a clinical trial. *Stat Med* 1992;**11**:23–35.

20 Spiegelhalter DJ, Freedman LS, Parmar MKB. Bayesian approaches to randomised trials. *J R Stat Soc* 1994;**157**:357–416.

21 Lilford RJ, Thornton JG, Braunholtz D. Clinical trials and rare diseases: a way out of a conundrum. *BMJ* 1995;**311**:1621–5.

22 Thornton JG, Lilford RJ, Johnson N. Decision analysis in medicine. *BMJ* 1992;**304**:1099–103.

23 Weinstein MC, Fineberg HV. *Clinical decision analysis.* London: Saunders, 1980.

24 Lilford RJ, Pauker SG, Braunholtz DA, Chard J. Decision analysis and the implementation of research findings. *BMJ* 1998;**317**:405–9.

25 Freedman B. Equipoise and ethics of clinical research. *N Engl J Med* 1987;**317**:141–5.

26 Johnson N, Lilford RJ, Brazier W. At what level of collective equipoise does a clinical trial become ethical? *J Med Ethics* 1991;**17**:30–4.

27 Gifford F. The conflict between randomised clinical trials and therapeutic obligation. *J Med Philos* 1986;**11**:347–66.

28 Kellett J, Clarke J. Comparison of "accelerated" tissue plasminogen activator with streptokinase for treatment of suspected myocardial infarction. *Med Decis Making* 1995;**15**:297–310.

29 Thornton JG, Lilford RJ. Decision analysis for medical managers. *BMJ* 1995;**310**:791–4.

30 Wragg JA, Robinson EJ, Lilford RJ. Information presentation and decisions to enter clinical trials: a hypothetical trial of hormone replacement therapy. *Soc Sci Med* 2000;**51**:453–62.

31 Edwards SJL, Lilford RJ, Braunholtz DA, Thornton J, Jackson J, Hewison J. Ethical issues in the design and conduct of randomised controlled trials. *Health Technol Assess* 1998;**2**:1–96.

32 Braunholtz DA, Edwards SJ, Lilford RJ. Are randomised clinical trials good for us (in the short term)? Evidence for a "trial effect". *J Clin Epidemiol* 2001;**54**:217–24.

33 Anonymous. Randomised trial of endarterectomy for recently symptomatic carotid stenosis: final results of the MRC European Carotid Surgery Trial (ECST). *Lancet* 1998;**351**:1379–87.

34 Edwards SJ, Lilford RJ, Braunholtz D, Jackson J. Why "under-powered" trials are not necessarily unethical. *Lancet* 1997;**350**: 804–7.

35 Fayers PM, Machin D. Sample size: how many patients are necessary? *Br J Cancer* 1995;**72**:1–9.

36 Freedman LS. The size of clinical trials in cancer research – what are the current needs? Medical Research Council Cancer Therapy Committee. *Br J Cancer* 1989;**59**:396–400.

11 "Empowering" patient choice about participation in trials?

HAZEL THORNTON

When I was given this title of "Empowering patient choice about participation in trials" I very nearly rejected it. Instead I turned it into a question,[1] and put inverted commas around the word "empowering". It is not a word I am very happy with, and have seldom used. *The Chambers Dictionary* defines it as: "the giving to individuals of power to take decisions in matters relating to themselves, esp. (in an organisation) in relation to self-development". My doubts may have been because I am more interested in considering the balance of power, rather than being given it.[2]

It has, however, made me realise that I must not be squeamish about this notion of "empowerment" if the problems of achieving good quality research that will *really* be of benefit to patients, as they see it, are to be addressed. As Iain Chalmers identified recently,[3] we need to find ways of enabling special interest patient groups, perhaps by using frameworks such as the *meta*Register of Current Controlled Trials, already in place on the internet,[4] to contribute to redressing the balance of power. This would help redirect research efforts where they are most needed, ultimately to provide most benefit and patient satisfaction with least wastage and optimum use of resources.[3]

I do believe in people being encouraged to take the initiative and behave as citizens with a right to challenge the status quo. This can be quite difficult in the world of medical research which has historically been viewed as a closed world of experts not open to "outsiders",[2] who intrude at their own peril. The population medical researchers used were referred to as "subjects", indeed still are in recent British Medical Journal *Education and Debate* papers,[5,6] conveying a notion of subjugation to kingly edicts. My own contrasting vision[7] was of iteration and negotiation, with participants making contributions of value to improve the quality of research and its usefulness to people, in company with various other kinds of experts. This would ensure that efforts were put into projects of relevance to the user, over and above the scientist. The shareholder, or the trustee.

"'Empowering' patient choice about participation in trials?" itself raised a host of questions in my mind around ownership, and the rights and responsibilities of either giving or receiving power in research endeavors. "Patient choice" is inanimate and cannot itself be empowered. How might "power to choose" be accomplished? What exactly is meant by "participation" in trials? As I see it, there are two kinds of patient participation in trials: active patient participation in research activities; and passive patient participation as participants in trials. If trials are for everyone – as we are all likely to be patients eventually, if not now – then they should, as Iain Chalmers has said, be "everyone's business".[8] And if they are "everyone's business", we are all stakeholders in the enterprise of conducting research. If so, it follows that we all, patients included, have an equal responsibility to see that there is fair play, and to challenge authority if we identify shortcomings.[9] Consumers are equally responsible, with everyone else, to work towards achieving a balance of power that will encourage the type of health care research that will enable choices. These would be choices made on the basis of reliable evidence, that citizens themselves identify as being important as they attempt to make decisions about their own health, or disease, management. And, if we are equally responsible, we should all be alert to circumstances, stratagems, legislation, and borderline or fraudulent practices[10–13] that threaten the main endeavour of improvement in health care for people which might thwart in any way research that will lead to users' satisfaction with methods, interventions and outcomes they seek and that matter to them.

We should also recognise that consumers are at a disadvantage by not only not having access, but by being denied access, even in apparently collaborative undertakings, to material that they need in order to be able to act on an equal footing with the other parties. For example, how can they judge whether a patient information sheet is a true reflection of a trial if they are denied access to the protocol? Also, how can anyone know if the participants have been presented with a fair and accurate portrayal of the research question and its implications, if the patient information leaflet is not provided or posted up with the protocol? How can reviewers of protocols, be they for funders or journals, or reviewers of reports of trials presented for publication, know if there have been ethical shortcomings in the consent process if the patient information sheet is not provided? They will not be able to judge if there has been inadequate or inaccurate portrayal of the trial to prospective participants to obtain agreement to their crucial part as partners in production of data. That is assuming the patient information sheet has actually been *given* to the patient![11] As Marilynn Larkin wrote, 'What price progress?' if drug companies' monetary incentives result in "short-cutting" the consent process? The patient information sheet should be the shop window of the trial, visible to all-comers, and accurately reflect the contents of the shop – perhaps with *Caveat emptor* inscribed over the entrance and *Caveat actor* over the exit?

Maintenance of equilibrium of any kind, be it physical or within societal endeavours, requires the constant outpouring of energy. In the research world, pressures from the burgeoning commercial research sector on the demand for trial participants for drug trials[10,11] makes it even more imperative that members of the lay public rise to the challenge. They will need to sharpen their critical faculties and address the problem, together with the help of clinical investigators, and involved organisations within and without the National Health Service. Consumers, after all "are likely to have the most unconflicted vested interests in promoting important trials".[3] They must not wait to be "empowered" but, as the citizens for whom this activity is supposedly being undertaken, contribute their arguments and ideas as of right.

This requires mutual encouragement. Patients can take action by throwing their drugs down the drain, or by voiding their inhalers into the air in trials of inhalants – to then be accused of cheating and "non-compliance". But it would be more constructive, less expensive, and produce more reliable data, to listen to their reasons for "non-compliance". A commentary by a special interest patients' group posted against such a trial on the web-based *meta*Register would provide illuminating food for thought both for trialists and potential participants. This alternative interpretation would allow readers to draw their own conclusions according to their own needs, values and judgement, empowering them to choose, enabling them to vote with their feet.[14] This approach would also promote the unpalatable truth that there is always uncertainty. Involving them in future research in that area would be likely to produce trial questions and trial protocols that would lead to evaluation of interventions that addressed patients' ideas of satisfaction. This presupposes a more "grown-up" dialogue[15] and, as Angela Coulter advocated, non-hierarchical partnerships that share responsibility and decision making, which recognise the expertise of patients. Unsatisfactory attempts at imposing solutions, as can frequently be seen, result in wastage of drugs, wastage of time, wastage of resources both human and financial, and production of severely contaminated data. What is required is: a pooling of ideas; a respect for the different kinds of expertise; a facing up to reality by both trialists and patients; and a proper motivation by all parties to be truly seeking the good of the patient. This is a total departure from the "them and us" culture, the "outsiders and insiders" culture in research, and research motivated, driven and perhaps dominated by commercial or other professional interests.[12,13]

Easier said than done, as we all know. Particularly when, as Richard Horton and Richard Smith in suggesting why it was "Time to register randomised trials"[16] said: "The process is chaotic". An attitudinal shift is required in many quarters.

An analysis by Mary Dixon-Woods: "Writing wrongs: an analysis of published discourses about the use of patient information leaflets"[17] identifies and describes the attitudinal problems beautifully. The analysis considers two contrasting discourses each revealing its own motivation for providing information to patients and the resultant mode and framing of that information. As she says: "the first .... derives its interest in printed information not from an imperative for democratisation, but from a concern with how communication might affect outcomes defined as biomedically important. The second discourse shows evidence of engagement with sociology and the social sciences, and much of its motivation for exploring the use of printed information comes from its interest in the role of information materials in (in inverted commas!) 'empowering' patients." The first discourse offers the pervasive view of patients as "irrational, passive, forgetful and incompetent". The second discourse depicts "a view of patients as competent, rational and resourceful, and engaged in continuous processes of meaning creation". The attitude and motivation of the information provider thus influences the framing of that information. It is plain that any debate involving both lay and professional is heavily dependent not only on the content and framing, but also on the motivation of those who have provided it.[18] One of the tenets of good information provision today is that consumers should be partners in its production. This is only part of the problem, as Julian Wragg, Elizabeth Robinson, and Richard Lilford have demonstrated in a study.[19] This showed that the same content in a patient information leaflet for a hypothetical trial of hormone replacement therapy, presented in what they labelled either "explicit" form or "ambiguous" form, resulted in different refusal rates. Or should I have framed it "acceptance" rates, seeing that this positive or negative reporting will resonate with, and affect your view, and remembrance, one way or the other![20]

The production of evidence to sift the harmful from the beneficial currently depends on those prepared to engage in it, and to do so in the face of onerous regulations designed to protect patients' rights. But is it right, one might ask, as I did, that those who governed the process to produce *Guidelines for Researchers*[21] to regulate that part of the profession seeking to improve the quality of health care, can impose this on them without consulting them, and can ignore the other part of the profession who choose not to participate in trials? Particularly as it is laid down that evidence-based health care is required by the National Health Service. Who has challenged the fairness of their process? Is it right that they can select those whom they consult, and decline to answer questions about the process of consultation they engaged in to produce the guidelines? Who empowered them to be guardians only of patients' rights, thereby widening divisions, doing little to foster trust or encourage critical collaboration? Who shall be guardian of the research community that seeks fair ways of evaluating health care interventions?[22]

I am astonished, and somewhat depressed, how ethical discussions seem to disregard the huge strides that have been made towards democratisation of research and inclusion of users' voices. "Research subjects" are discussed as though they were one homogeneous, passive, entity, largely incompetent, mostly vulnerable, in need of protection, without a voice of their own. But research today is global: systematic reviews attempt to be global; the *meta*Register of Current Controlled Trials[4] is international. But the increasingly wide search for participants by industry, sometimes through contract research organisations, widens the net to the most vulnerable and gullible people, both in highly developed nations like the United States of America and undeveloped countries. However much we might need and enjoy debates about equipoise and uncertainty, action is needed in the face of dubious, serious protocol violations exposed in seven US research institutions,[10] or the dishonest stratagems identified by Marilynn Larkin,[12] corroborated anecdotally in my own experience.

But optimism wins when I consider the efforts being made by the Cochrane Collaboration to incorporate consumers in the fight to raise the quality of research. Other institutions in the United Kingdom have also identified the value of consumers working together with health care professionals to better balance the scales to achieve better quality, relevant, appropriate research. As Paul Dieppe and colleagues of the Medical Research Council Health Services Research Collaboration stated: "Industrial funding of trials has undue influence on the research agenda and distorts the body of published evidence. Healthcare professionals need to work with consumers to decide what intervention research is of most value to patients, and then to look for ways of funding pivotal trials in these areas, rather than playing along with the agenda of the pharmaceutical industry".[23] They cite a review and their own focus group work with sufferers of osteoarthritis of the knee, which demonstrated that stakeholders thought that the priorities of the current drug research for that condition were inappropriate.[24] The review identified 509 trials, 414 of which (81%) were drug trials. The stakeholders felt that there should be more work on physical, surgical, and educational interventions.

Today, knowledge management is a skill. Acquisition of that skill is but one aspect. Utilisation of that knowledge for the good of man is a more difficult problem. Cultural and attitudinal barriers remain aplenty. The pace of technological developments is out-stripping our ability to properly and adequately consider and develop the ethics. What lies at the very heart of making sense of knowledge, our attitudes to it, and ultimately our ethical stances, is: the need for different, but equally valid interpretations[14]; challenges to deliberately misrepresented or manipulated historical evidence or data[25]; enablement of "meaning creation"[16] derived from good quality information materials; and appreciation of the use of different methods of presentation of the same information to achieve specific results.[17]

References

1 Editor's Choice. Answers descend, questions ascend. *BMJ* 2000;**321**:A.
2 Refractor. "Insiders" and "outsiders" in research collaborations? *Lancet* 2000;**356**:1038.
3 Chalmers I. A patient-led *Good Controlled Trials Guide*. *Lancet* 2000;**356**:774.

4 Current Controlled Trials. www.controlled-trials.com (accessed 11 Jul 2001).

5 Rothman KJ, Michels KB, Baum M. Education and Debate. For and against: Declaration of Helsinki should be strengthened. *BMJ* 2000;**321**:442–5.

6 Thornton H. Response to: For and against: Declaration of Helsinki should be strengthened. *eBMJ* 15 Aug 2000. www.bmj.com/cgi/eletters/321/7258/442#EL5 (accessed 11 Jul 2001).

7 Thornton H. The patient's role in research. In: *Health Committee Third Report: Breast Cancer Services*. Vol. ll. London: HMSO 1995: 113–4.

8 Chalmers I, Silverman WA. Professional and public double standards on clinical experimentation. *Control Clin Trials* 1987;**8**: 388–91.

9 Silverman WA, Chalmers I. Casting and drawing lots. In: Chalmers I, Milne I, Douglas S, eds. *Controlled Trials from History*. www.rcpe.ac.uk/controlled trials (accessed 21 Aug 2000).

10 Editorial. Safeguarding participants in clinical trials. *Lancet* 2000; **355**:2177.

11 Horton R. Commentary. The less acceptable face of bias. *Lancet* 2000; **356**:959–60.

12 Larkin M. Clinical Trials: what price progress? *Lancet* 1999; **354**:1534.

13 Thornton H. Relationship of trial design to value of data for patient? *Eur J Cancer* 2000;**36**:1585–6.

14 Thornton H. Clinical trials, consensus conferences, and clinical practice. *Lancet* 1999;**354**:1037.

15 Coulter A. Paternalism or partnership? *BMJ* 1999;**319**:719–20.

16 Horton R, Smith R. Time to register randomised trials. *BMJ* 1999; **319**:865–6.

17 Dixon-Woods M. Writing wrongs? An analysis of published discourses about the use of patient information leaflets. *Soc Sci Med* 2001; **52**:1417–32.

18 Thornton, H. What's it like to be talked to? *SCAN* 2000;**11**:42–3.

19 Wragg JA, Robinson EJ, Lilford RJ. Information presentation and decision to enter clinical trials: a hypothetical trial of hormone replacement therapy. *Soc Sci Med* 2000;**51**:453–62.

20 Tversky A, Kahneman D. The framing of decisions and psychology of choice. *Science* 1981;**211**:453–8.

21 Guidelines for Researchers: Patient Information Sheet and Consent Form. The Scottish Office, Department of Health. (Ref: SDS0210M) April 1999.

22 Refractor. "Guardianship". *Lancet* 2001;**357**:1808.

23 Dieppe P, Chard J, Tallon D, Egger M. Funding clinical research. *Lancet* 1999;**353**:1626.

24 Chard JA, Tallon D, Dieppe PA. Epidemiology of research into interventions for the treatment of osteoarthritis of the knee joint. *Ann Rheum Dis* 2000;59:414–18.
25 Irving HM. The Verdict. Judge delivers a devastating condemnation. *The Times*. April 12 2000: *News*: 7.

Index

Page numbers in **bold** refer to figures; those in *italic* refer to tables or boxed material